Providing Acute Care

EELCO F. M. WIJDICKS, M.D., PH.D.,FACP, FNCS, FANA
Professor of Neurology, Mayo Clinic College of Medicine
Chair, Division of Critical Care Neurology
Consultant, Neurosciences Intensive Care Unit
Saint Marys Hospital
Mayo Clinic, Rochester, Minnesota

OXFORD
PRESS

D1207799

OXFORD
UNIVERSITY PRESS

Oxford University Press is a department of the University of Oxford.
It furthers the University's objective of excellence in research, scholarship,
and education by publishing worldwide.

Oxford   New York
Auckland   Cape Town   Dar es Salaam   Hong Kong   Karachi
Kuala Lumpur   Madrid   Melbourne   Mexico City   Nairobi
New Delhi   Shanghai   Taipei   Toronto

With offices in
Argentina   Austria   Brazil   Chile   Czech Republic   France   Greece
Guatemala   Hungary   Italy   Japan   Poland   Portugal   Singapore
South Korea   Switzerland   Thailand   Turkey   Ukraine   Vietnam

Oxford is a registered trademark of Oxford University Press
in the UK and certain other countries.

Published in the United States of America by
Oxford University Press
198 Madison Avenue, New York, NY 10016

© Oxford University Press 2014

Library of Congress Cataloging-in-Publication Data
Wijdicks, Eelco F. M., 1954– author.
Providing acute care / Eelco F.M. Wijdicks.
    p. ; cm.—(Core principles of acute neurology)
Includes bibliographical references.
ISBN 978–0–19–992875–0 (alk. paper)
I. Title.   II. Series: Core principles of acute neurology.
[DNLM: 1. Acute Disease–therapy.   2. Nervous System Diseases—therapy.
3. Critical Care—methods.   4. Hospitalists—methods.   5. Nervous System
Diseases—complications. WL 140]
RA975.5.R47
616.2'0046—dc23
2013029347

9 8 7 6 5 4 3 2 1
Printed in the United States of America
on acid-free paper

For Barbara, Coen, and Marilou

Contents

Preface

The medical care of hospitalized neurologic patients can be fairly simple, particularly in patients admitted to be prepared for surgery or in patients admitted for thorough evaluation of a neurodegenerative disorder. However, hospitalized acutely ill neurologic patients may have major medical problems or develop them shortly after admission.

This book thus concentrates on medical problems that are often puzzling and worrisome. Many of these medical problems may become severe enough to warrant transfer to a monitored bed or formidable enough to go to an ICU. Often these medical problems are part of daily care. Any neurologist or resident in neurology taking care of acutely hospitalized patients should have a good foundation of knowledge of other medical specialties, but without crossing boundaries and assuming unwanted responsibilities.

How do we keep the patient medically stable and what do we check every day? How do we prevent infections and when do we treat with antibiotics? What antibiotics do we use? How do we manage hyperglycemia? How do we interpret laboratory derangements and correct them? How do we manage anticoagulation or prevent thrombotic complications? What drug side effects and drug-drug interactions should we be familiar with? Surprisingly little information on the nitty gritty of daily care in the acutely ill neurologic patient can be found in current hospitalist books. This volume will have a major focus on how certain neurologic conditions can inflict damage to other organ systems and what systemic complications most frequently jeopardize patients with primary neurological disorders. This book may assist any resident and fellow—writing the orders and on the front line—but also any hospitalists, neurohospitalists, and neurointensivists in their daily medical care.

Introduction to the Series

The confrontation with an acutely ill neurologic patient is quite an unsettling situation for physicians, but all will have to master how to manage the patient at presentation, how to shepherd the unstable patient to an intensive care unit, and how to take charge. To do that aptly, knowledge of the principles of management is needed. Books on the clinical practice of acute, emergency and critical care neurology have appeared, but none have yet treated the fundamentals in depth.

Core Principles of Acute Neurology is a series of short volumes that handles topics not found in sufficient detail elsewhere. The books focus precisely on those areas that require a good working knowledge. These are: the consequences of acute neurologic diseases, medical care in all its aspects and relatedness with the injured brain, difficult decisions in complex situations. Because the practice involves devastatingly injured patients, there is a separate volume on prognostication and neuropalliation. Other volumes are planned in the future.

The series has unique features. I hope to contextualize basic science with clinical practice in a readable narrative with a light touch and without wielding the jargon of this field. The ten chapters in each volume try to spell out in the clearest terms how things work. The text is divided into a description of principles followed by its relevance to practice— keeping it to the bare essentials. There are boxes inserted into the text with quick reminders ("By the Way") and useful percentages carefully researched and vetted for accuracy ("By the Numbers"). Drawings are used to illustrate mechanisms and pathophysiology.

These books cannot cover an entire field, but brevity and economy allows a focus on one topic at a time. Gone are the days of large, doorstop tomes with many words on paper but with little practical value. This series is therefore characterized by simplicity—in a good sense—and it is acute and critical care neurology at the core, not encyclopedic but representative. I hope it supplements clinical curricula or comprehensive textbooks.

The audience is primarily neurologists and neurointensivists, neurosurgeons, fellows, and residents. Neurointensivists have increased in numbers, and many major institutions have attendings and fellowship programs. However, these books cross disciplines and should also be useful for intensivists, anesthesiologists, emergency physicians, nursing staff, and allied health care professionals in intensive care units and the emergency department. In the end the intent is to write a book that provides a sound reassuring basis to practice well, and that helps with understanding and appreciating the complexities of care of a patient with an acute neurologic condition.

1

An Acute Care Plan

The call comes: "The patient is here." Dealing with an acutely ill neurologic patient, whether in the emergency department, neurology ward, or intensive care unit (ICU), carries a tense immediacy for any physician. The diagnosis may be known—at least up to a certain point—but after the "ABCs" are checked, where to start? The reasonable, comfortable notion of being able to care for any medically ill patient is not sufficient when it comes to acutely ill neurologic patients, and the line of thinking in neurologic disease is vastly different from that in other medical disciplines. One misjudgment can set off a cascade of problems, easily leading to a more serious condition. One is reminded of the mildly breathless patient with myasthenia gravis and perfect arterial blood gases who late at night develops a respiratory arrest and ends up with permanent anoxic-ischemic brain injury. Acute neurologic illness may initially divert attention from medical comorbidities that may flare up during hospitalization. Underappreciating the potential for major medical complications in an acutely ill neurologic patient thus may lead to higher risk of mortality (Figure 1.1).[1,10,17]

Physicians must go through a set of assessments, verifications, and decisions that ultimately stabilize or treat the patient with an acute neurologic disease. How is that done effectively? How is one to judge acute situations appropriately and with common sense? This opening chapter provides a systems approach adjusted for the acutely ill neurologic patient, wherever seen in the hospital, and helps to prioritize.

Principles

The care of an acutely ill neurologic patient begins with several essential—and often recurring—questions.

Attending physicians have to decide whether they are competent in resuscitating patients without the assistance of their peers. Every physician should know what his or her boundaries are. Physicians confident in their skills should not hesitate to intervene; those who are uncertain should seek help from colleagues. Most hospital practices are currently able to activate a "rapid response team."[2,12,15,21,23]

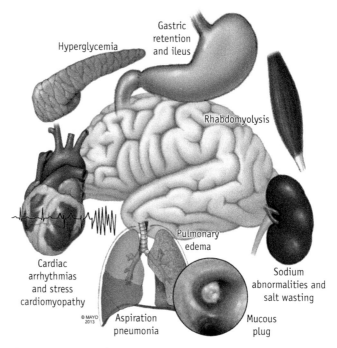

Figure 1.1 Major anticipated medical complications after acute brain injury

These rapid response calls have taught physicians warning signs that especially apply to neurologic patients. It often involves an obstructed airway, any sense of respiratory difficulty, breathing less than 10 breaths/min or more than 28 breaths/min, and pulse oximeter saturation <90%.[3] Furthermore, acute chest pain, a compromised circulation with a pulse less than 40 bpm or more than 120 bpm, hypotension measured as a systolic blood pressure less than 90 mm Hg, and the observation of a poor urinary output of less than 20 mL/hour are all warning signs and indications for transfer to an intensive care unit.

IS ACUTE INTUBATION NEEDED?

Assessment of airway comes first, but somehow its tremendous importance in acute neurologic conditions is not always fully acknowledged. Upper airway obstruction may be initially relieved by removal of dentures and reopening of the airway by so-called head tilt/chin lift—an often forgotten maneuver—as tilting the head back to the sniff position improves the trachea/pharynx angulation. The index and middle finger of the examiner's hand also lifts the mandible, which brings the tongue forward.

Intubation in obese patients requires specific attention. Some techniques include "ramped" position (head and shoulders elevated above chest), CPAP preoxygenation and dosing of succinylcholine according to total body weight.[5] An oropharyngeal airway can often be placed and is particularly useful to maintain an open airway. It may also prevent tongue biting, which is of particular importance if seizures have been suspected. Patients may need to be "bagged" and transported to an ICU for intubation. Indications for intubation have been well established and includes any patient who demonstrates a decreased responsiveness and marginal oxygenation, any patient who is tachypneic, tachycardic, or has increased effort of breathing, and any patient who displays wheezing or stridor.

In patients with acute neuromuscular disease, intubation is required for patients with hypoventilation and hypoxia. Myasthenia gravis, Guillain-Barré syndrome (GBS), and amyotrophic lateral sclerosis (ALS) are commonly seen in the emergency department. Examination of patients with breathlessness due to neuromuscular disease should focus on oropharyngeal dysfunction, impaired coughing, and paradoxical (abdominal) breathing. Patients with an acutely progressive disorder (e.g., GBS) may not have enough muscular reserve to breathe satisfactorily with a pressure-support mode (BiPAP) and may need full mechanical ventilation after intubation.

The symptoms and signs of acute neuromuscular respiratory failure are subtle. In some patients paradoxical (thoracoabdominal asynchrony) breathing is seen with abdomen moving in and chest out.[27] Many patients have staccato speech and a need to pause after a few words. Sweat is often found at the hairline or collects in the eyebrows and is a sign of the increased effort of breathing. Restlessness may be apparent, but some patients are quiet and simply nod "yes" when asked if they are short of breath. Passage of air through the nose when asked to blow up the cheek against counterpressure by the examiner's thumb and index finger can be seen and reveals additional oropharyngeal weakness. The assessment of oropharyngeal weakness implies not only that respiratory mechanics could be involved but also that ineffective swallowing could lead to aspiration.

Intubation in the emergency department has evolved into a standardized approach also known as "rapid sequence intubation."[9,18,19] The sequence has been remembered by the "6 P's" (preparation, preoxygenation, premedication, paralysis, and postintubation care). The rapid sequence is the near-simultaneous administration of an induction agent and a paralytic agent. One physician prepares the patient for intubation, placing the patient in Trendelenburg position, gathering the intubation blade, and setting up the mechanical ventilator. The other administers the drugs in sequence, having all syringes identified and lined up. When a drug is administered, the physician mentions the dose and drug to the team. The pretreatment phase attenuates the physiologic response during intubation, and preinduction drugs (lidocaine, esmolol, or opioids) have been used, but strictly speaking, there is little evidence for their effectiveness. About three minutes later the induction phase begins, and the agents rapidly cause unconsciousness. After mask ventilation with an inspiratory pressure of 10–12 cm water, the following agents are typically administered: (1) preinduction agents—midazolam 20 mg IV and fentanyl 50 mcg IV push; (2) induction agents—etomidate 20 mg IV push or ketamine 100 mg IV push; and (3) paralytic agents—succinylcholine 70 mg IV push or rocuronium 50 mg IV push. Succinylcholine is contraindicated in chronic muscular disease because of the risk of hyperkalemia, but this complication is neither common nor always lifethreatening. The initial setting on the mechanical ventilator is "assist control" to provide adequate ventilation while patients are undergoing tests or if hyperventilation is needed. This will also prevent unexpected hypoxemia and hypercapnia if the patient does not ventilate well. The patient can be transitioned to SIMV/pressure support ventilation when in a more secure environment. Tidal volumes should be 6 mL/kg ideal (and not true) bodyweight, but in obese patients this may still be insufficient and lead to ventilator dyssynchrony. Increasing tidal volume or flow or better a fentanyl infusion will alleviate this concern.

IS CIRCULATION ADEQUATE?

Assessment of circulation comes next or simultaneously. Fluid resuscitation is necessary in many neurologic patients who are dehydrated due to absence of thirst. Immediate intravenous access with a large-bore catheter is needed to provide a crystalloid, usually 500 mL of normal saline, to see an initial response (more is likely needed).[25,29] Albumin can be administered if the patient is in shock, but it is less rapidly available. Any resuscitation cart should have a phenylephrine syringe that can be used to administer 200 mcg in a single dose that will improve blood pressure quickly before the patient is transported to the ICU. Repeated pushes may be needed until central access is secured.

IS THE PATIENT ACTIVELY SEIZING?

Unresponsive patients might be actively seizing. It is clinically impossible to differentiate between nonconvulsive status epilepticus and a prolonged postictal state. Forced gaze and eyelid or extremity twitching are not often seen because they are fleeting and gone by the time the physician arrives. Most patients display marked fluctuations in lucidity, with moments of eye contact and responsiveness followed by eyelid closure, twitching, and eye deviation. Some patients are drowsy and have rhythmic jaw or hand twitches. An EEG will determine an ictal (rhythmic sharp waves) or interictal (periodic generalized epileptiform discharges) state.

Protecting the patient from harm during seizures—padding in bed—is an essential part of resuscitation. The administration of intravenous antiepileptic agents is problematic on the ward. If necessary (while awaiting arrival of antiepileptic drugs), 4 to 8 mg of lorazepam can be easily administered on the ward without significantly compromising respiration. One single IV dose of 4 mg lorazepam may "wake up" the patient rapidly and can be almost as impressive as correcting hypoglycemia.

DO I NEED MORE TESTS?

Three neurologic tests—CT scanning and magnetic resonance imaging (MRI), CSF examination, and electroencephalogram—should be immediately available and may substantially narrow the diagnostic evaluation. CT scan and computed tomographic angiogram (CTA)—or MRI and magnetic resonance angiogram (MRA)—of the brain may be required for timely evaluation in an emergency involving the central nervous system, but CSF examination and electroencephalography are needed with certain clinical suspicions. Important dilemmas appear when the CT scan does not fit the patient's neurologic finding or is normal. The yield of an MRI is substantially higher and may provide an answer in evolving encephalitis (particularly limbic and herpes simplex), anoxic-ischemic injury, posterior reversible encephalopathy syndrome, cerebritis, epidural empyema, and ischemic stroke in the posterior circulation. A stat MRI should be carefully considered, and a convincing rationale will have to be provided to the radiologist. CTA (or MRA) and computed tomographic venography (CTV) or magnetic resonance venography (MRV) are underutilized but may help diagnose acute arterial or venous occlusions, or arterial vasospasm, as in cerebral vasoconstriction syndrome.

Any patient with a severe head injury (and certainly patients on anticoagulation or with a coagulopathy) may need a follow-up CT scan to look for blossoming contusions or developing subdural hematomas. Any patient with a head injury due to fall a CT of the cervical spine (possibly MRI and later flexion and extension images.)

Very few blood tests are immediately helpful in patients with an established neurologic diagnosis, but they are needed to assess the general medical condition. A set of complete blood count, electrolytes, liver and kidney function tests, thyroid-stimulating hormone (TSH), ammonia, and arterial blood gas may provide initial useful information, and often reassurance, before moving on to further diagnostic tests.

IS THE PATIENT IN THE RIGHT PLACE AND AT RISK FOR DETERIORATION?

Patients with acute neurologic injury can be seen anywhere and may need to be transferred to the ICU or at least a monitored bed. The risk of neurologic deterioration will have to be assessed immediately. Approximately 10%–20% of patients are inappropriately admitted to the ward after an acute neurologic injury and may deteriorate within hours after presentation. Any worsening of neurologic condition could prompt transfer to an ICU or, preferably, a neurosciences intensive care unit (NICU).

Criteria for ICU admission can be established by ICU directors and as expected will include any patient with a deteriorating neurologic deficit, need for intravenous sedation in agitation, concern about respiratory support in a comatose patient, refractory seizures, cardiac arrhythmias or abnormal troponin, and refractory hypertension or hypotension. A patient with an acute neurologic disease should be considered unstable and many aspects of medical care require immediate attention.

IS WHAT I SEE EXPECTED WHEN I LOOK AT THE PATIENT?

Patients may not "look as advertised." This requires neurologic expertise, and getting a feel for it requires years of being exposed to these problems. Commonly the patient is less responsive than what is expected based on initial CT scan results. The CT scan may show a small lesion with mass effect or may even be normal. In these patients a repeat CT scan will be revealing, and it almost always will involve patients with severe traumatic brain injury developing new contusions with mass effect or patients with expanding cerebral hematomas in patients previously treated with warfarin. Undocumented anoxia or prior cardiopulmonary resuscitation may explain a comatose patient with a normal CT scan. In some patients there is an acute laboratory abnormality or there is a developing multisystem illness with rapidly changing laboratory parameters. A new full set of laboratory tests may be needed.

IS AN IMMEDIATE NEUROSURGICAL INTERVENTION NEEDED?

One has to determine early on whether neurosurgical consult is needed and whether an intervention can be anticipated. These are not situations that are "perhaps" or "probably." Urgent neurosurgical indications are often obvious at the time of arrival, usually involving the presence of an acute mass effect and brain tissue displacement. The presence of an acute subdural or epidural hematoma is a neurosurgical emergency that often requires evacuation. Any cerebral lesion with mass effect may immediately require decompression. Indications for acute—the same day or night—craniotomy or craniectomy depends on neurologic condition at presentation. Only the presence of pathologic flexion or extensor motor responses and absence of several brainstem reflexes as a result of pontomesencephalic damage may suggest that neurosurgical intervention is not indicated. However in cerebellar lesions these clinical signs may not necessarily indicate poor outcome because they may indicate brainstem compression that can be relieved with surgery.

In any patient with a cerebral hematoma, the question is whether the patient is actively bleeding. Patients on warfarin immediately need vitamin K, fresh frozen plasma, and, because of the urgency and the possibility of surgery, an appropriate dose of recombinant activated factor VII (40 mcg/kg) or prothrombin complex concentrate (varies but usually 30–40 units/kg). Prothrombin complex concentrate has been recommended as a preferred treatment (Chapter 8).

Any comatose patient with a new displacing mass is at high risk of increasing intracranial pressure (ICP) and belongs in an ICU. Most major trauma centers use a fiber-optic intraparenchymal device that measures ICP. An intraparenchymal ICP monitor provides not only an ICP value but also the cerebral perfusion pressure (CPP), which can be calculated knowing the mean arterial blood pressure

(MAP). The abbreviated formula is CCP=MAP – ICP. The optimal ICP and CPP are currently defined as an ICP less than 20 mm Hg and a CPP between 50 and 70 mm Hg (see volume on recognizing brain injury for more detailed discussion).

Treatment of increased intracranial pressure first requires aggressive oxygenation and correction of hypercarbia followed by hyperventilation (arterial PCO_2 in the 30s) and administration of 20% mannitol using a full bolus of 1 g/kg. The use of hypertonic saline (any concentration of 3% or more) requires the placement of a central venous catheter, and waiting for that to be in place could markedly delay initial treatment of ICP. Moreover, putting the patient flat or in slight Trendelenburg position to place a central catheter is not advised as it may cause an ICP surge. Therefore, mannitol first, central line next, followed by repeated doses of hypertonic saline.

To establish unsuccessful ICP control may take some time, but rapid review of possible modifiable factors such fever, seizures, agitation, hypercarbia, or hypoxemia (with high positive end-expiratory pressure, or PEEP) is warranted. Any proven unsuccessful control of ICP will have to be treated with decompressive craniectomy or removal of a bone flap if it follows prior evacuation of a contusion or extracranial hematoma. The initial experience with decompressive craniectomy has shown significant reduction in ICP surges, and delay in contacting and convincing a neurosurgeon to proceed may have consequences for the patient's potential for recovery or, in extreme cases, there may be further deterioration.

Failure to recognize acute hydrocephalus is common in any acute emergency. For example, in subarachnoid hemorrhage the focus may be on the hemorrhage, which is thought to explain the clinical condition, but acute cerebrospinal fluid (CSF) obstruction from intraventricular blood or from heavy clot burden in the cisterns may lead to reduced level of consciousness. This can quickly be treated with placement of a ventriculostomy. Not infrequently, CSF pours out under high pressure after puncture of the frontal horn.

On another note, urgency may also involve acute spinal cord disorders. The approach to acute spinal cord compression is determined by its cause, but immediate surgical management is a much-needed approach in patients with an epidural abscess localized at a few levels, epidural hematoma, or extradural metastasis with rapidly evolving neurologic deterioration. Its benefit lies in preservation of at least partial mobility and, equally important, complete bladder function. In cases of patients with acute spinal cord compression, rapid decision-making is paramount because reversal of tetraparesis or paraparesis becomes less likely with passing of time. If vertebral collapse coincides with spinal cord compression, the chances for ambulation are lower. Dexamethasone is given to all patients with metastatic cord compression (100 mg IV push followed by 16 mg/day PO in divided doses) until definitive management has been determined. Surgery is also warranted when the primary tumor is unknown and histologic diagnosis is needed.

In Practice

Medical care usually proceeds through systems. This has been an effective way of organizing care, and it likely secures a comprehensive assessment. Most patients with an acute neurologic injury have other medical issues, which often may cause concerns in the days after admission. Neurologists have all seen worsening of congestive heart failure, new cardiac arrhythmias, poor control of diabetes mellitus, and unstable blood pressures. It is essential for the admitting neurologist to obtain information about past medical history, medication, allergies, and history of drug and alcohol use. In addition, it is important to obtain evidence of prior advanced dementia, which increases the risk of in-hospital delirium. It is even more important to obtain information about possible injury that may have occurred as a result of a fall.

The full medical physical examination that follows should include pulmonary evaluation with listening to breath sounds, cardiovascular status with confirmation of the patency of the peripheral vasculature, and full abdominal evaluation for possible tenderness and expansion. This initial evaluation is then immediately followed by a review of all known diagnostic studies,which should include a chest X-ray and an initial laboratory panel. A chest X-ray may have to be repeated if there is evidence of possible aspiration or other types of pulmonary injury. Joint X-rays may be necessary if the patient has seriously injured himself and bruises are obvious. Any patient with a fall, or who was found down helpless at home for an unknown time, should have creatinine kinase evaluated. Rhabdomyolysis with elevated serum muscle enzymes, including creatinine kinase, is associated with urine discoloration and may rapidly result in hyperkalemia and acute kidney injury.

Laboratory studies should include a complete blood count, renal function test, urea nitrogen, and creatinine, particularly in patients who have received intravenous contrast agents. A serum creatinine concentration usually rises within 24 hours of the contrast administration and may be associated with oliguria; it can evolve into a significant contrast-induced nephropathy (Chapter 10). Coagulation parameters, including platelets and international normalized ratio (INR), should be known before any neurosurgical intervention.

APPROACH BY SYSTEM

A system approach involves a careful look at organ systems and can be broadened to include common issues that emerge during hospital stay, such as infections, problems with intravenous access to the patient, and preventive measures with so-called bundles.

A common occurrence is delirium in an elderly patient with an acute neurologic disorder.[11,16] A useful tool is the confusion assessment method that specifically looks at acute onset or fluctuating course—and is usually obtained from a family member who may confirm that there has been acute change from the patient baseline—but also whether the patient's behavior seems to fluctuate throughout the day.[28] Noteworthy behavior includes difficulty focusing attention, easy distractibility or difficulty keeping track of what has been said, disorganized thinking with rambling conversation that includes illogical flow of ideas and unpredictable switching from subject to subject, and any altered level of consciousness that makes the patient difficult to arouse. A large proportion of patients with delirium have a so-called quiet delirium that needs to be recognized. Acute delirium may be related to an acute electrolyte imbalance, severe dehydration, or new-onset infection. Delirium can be treated, most of the time, with atypical antipsychotics. Benzodiazepine should be avoided unless delirium is caused by alcohol or benzodiazepine withdrawal. The atypical antipsychotics olanzapine or quetiapine are quite effective but may result in prolonged QT interval on EKG that may limit its use.[26] Severe agitation treatment would require admission to a more secure setting.

Oxygenation and respiratory rate are good measures and pulse oximeter may provide useful monitoring. Respiratory rate is a "neglected vital sign."[3] Acute new tachypnea should require evaluation for aspiration, hospital-acquired pneumonia and pulmonary emboli (Chapter 3). For uncertain situations a CT/CTA of the chest may be quite helpful.

Fluid administration is usually set at 50–70 mLof normal saline per hour. Dehydration is difficult to measure, and laboratory abnormalities such as hypernatremia and uremia are only seen in more severe causes of dehydration. Fluid administration should be guided by urinary production and measuring of fluid balance. Fluid and electrolyte replacement and maintenance are dependent on the dietary status and can be adjusted. Usually crystalloid boluses are administered in patients who are oligoric or who have developed a negative fluid balance. On the other hand, a positive fluid balance is often seen in patients who had significant fluid administration during transport, following which intake should be minimized. Electrolytes are replaced and have to be specifically checked for normalization. The electrolytes that are frequently measured are potassium, sodium, phosphate, and magnesium. Many patients have no ongoing renal issues except for some patients with chronic renal failure. As alluded to earlier, the risk of contrast-induced nephropathy is real in acute neurologic disease as a result of use of CT angiogram and other contrast studies. A risk score is found in Chapter 10.

Brainstem stroke in particular but any ischemic stroke increases the risk of aspiration.[8,20,22] Insular cortex involvement together with frontal lesions do seem to increase risk of aspiration.[6] The cough reflex is notoriously unreliable.[24] A bedside test for swallowing dysfunction is important, and aspiration to thin liquid resulting in spontaneous cough during test swallows increases the risk of aspiration greatly. Further evaluation of swallowing is necessary, but enteral nutrition may have to be started in patients with little reserve. Enteral feeding may significantly increase fluid intake, and the total fluid intake will have to be adjusted. Glucose control is important in both diabetic and nondiabetic patients. Generally, blood glucose is held between 140 and 180 mg/dL—better control will reduce the length of stay, mortality, and infection proclivity.

In ensuing days, infection is carefully monitored and is typically recognized by new-onset fever, increasing white blood cell count, and positive cultures. Infectious surveillance is important but can easily lead to overtreatment. Asymptomatic bacteriuria is found in approximately 50% of elderly admissions, and some patients may have antibiotic-resistant pathogens such as methacycline-resistant *Staphylococcus aureus* or vancomycin-resistant *Enterococi*. Appropriate isolation measures may be needed (Chapter 9).

Prophylaxis includes gastric ulcer prophylaxis. Patient should be on a proton pump inhibitor or H2 receptor antagonists, when mechanically ventilated or on high-dose corticosteroids. Prophylaxis for venous thrombosis requires intermittent calf compression devices in any patient. Its efficacy is proven in immobilized patients with a stroke.[4] Deep venous thrombosis prophylaxis is usually provided with subcutaneous heparin or low-molecular-weight heparin. In general, low-dose low-molecular-weight heparin, despite higher cost, offers the best benefit-to-risk ratio for prophylaxis of deep venous thrombosis and venous embolism, but most hospital practices peruse subcutaneous heparin.[13,14] Prophylactic heparin can be started (after 48 hours) in any patient with a recent intracerebral hemorrhage, any patient with a nonhemorrhagic brain tumor, any patient with traumatic brain injury, and any patient with recent central nervous system infection, but should be withheld in patients with unsecured ruptured aneurysm, ventriculostomy, or lumbar drain and soon after acute spine surgery. Surveillance with ultrasound studies is necessary—weekly in predisposed patients.

Access will have to be secured in most patients, and this is a peripheral venous access. When a transfer to the ICU is anticipated, a second access may be needed to facilitate the use of IV drugs. Patency of IV access is one of the most important items to check in a patient. A peripherally inserted central catheter (PICC) line, or internal jugular or subclavian catheter should be considered in patients who would require IV antibiotics or hypertonic solutions or when venous access cannot be guaranteed.

Code status—to resuscitate or not—will need to be determined and discussed with patient and family member. Such as discussion includes both escalation and deescalation of care and its criteria. This discussion may come very soon in the care of the patient particularly if the clinical situation seems hopeless.

The most important questions that must be asked during rounds are summarized in Table 1.1.

Table 1.1 **Items to Discuss During Rounds**

Mechanical Ventilation
➤ Settings ok? (TV 4–6 mg/kg PBW, Pplat <30 cm H$_2$O, PEEP <5 cm H$_2$O, SpO2 88%–95%)
➤ Can weaning be initiated? Review duration of MV. Should tracheostomy be considered?
➤ Head of bed elevation ≥30

Sedation and Analgesia
➤ Protocol ordered and sedation holidays?
➤ Options for nonopiate analgesics ordered?
➤ Pain control adequate?
➤ Alcohol withdrawal protocol initiated?
➤ Other steps for intervention ordered?

Fever
➤ Drugs or cooling device ordered?
➤ Defined temperature threshold ordered?

Antibiotics
➤ Need for antibiotics (culture positive or clinical judgment)?
➤ Culture sensitivities reviewed?
➤ Can antibiotics be narrowed?

Nutrition
➤ Days without nutrition, route, diet type, and target reviewed?
➤ Is a calorie count needed?
➤ Is a PEG tube required?
➤ Insulin drip reviewed? Targets appropriate?

Bowel Care
➤ Motility measures and drugs ordered?

Lines
➤ Indwelling catheters reviewed and dates placed?

Mobility
➤ Can activity orders be upgraded?
➤ Physical therapy has been ordered?

Skin Condition
➤ Reviewed with nursing and ordered therapy?

Venous Thrombosis and Stress Ulcer Prophylaxis
➤ Unfractionated or subcutaneous heparin or contraindication noted?
➤ Screening ultrasound in immobile patients every 5–7 days ordered?
➤ Indication of ulcer prophylaxis reviewed?

Code Status
➤ Is code status clear? Appropriate? Further discussions indicated?

By the Way

Potential for Deterioration
- Any mass lesion or tumor with edema
- Any spinal cord compression
- More than one seizure before transport
- Prior alcoholism
- Hypertension
- Cardiac arrhythmia and new atrial fibrillation

Acute Illness by the Numbers

- ~80% rapid response team admits to ICU
- ~75% deterioration on the ward due to sedation, seizures, or hypertension
- ~50% deterioration on the ward middle of the night
- ~50% deterioration antecedent concerns expressed
- ~30% reduction of cardiac arrest with rapid response team
- ~20% reduction of mortality with rapid response team

Putting It All Together

- Wrong triage of an acutely ill neurologic patient is common
- Medically stable patients may be neurologically unstable and vice versa
- Many patients with acute neurologic disease deteriorate from sedation and opioid overuse
- In patients with an unclear neurologic presentation one must secure an ICU bed
- Level of care and resuscitation status should be discussed early

References

1. Bae HJ, Yoon DS, Lee J, et al. In-hospital medical complications and long-term mortality after ischemic stroke. *Stroke* 2005;36:2441.
2. Chan PS, Jain R, Nallmothu BK, Berg RA, Sasson C. Rapid response teams: a systematic review and meta-analysis. *Arch Intern Med* 2010;170:18–26.
3. Cretikos MA, Bellomo R, Hillman K, et al. Respiratory rate: the neglected vital sign. *Med J Aust* 2008;188:657–659.
4. CLOTS (Clots in Legs Or sTockings after Stroke) Trials Collaboration. Dennis M, Sandercock P. Reid J, Graham C, Forbes J, Murray G. Effectiveness of intermittent pneumatic compression in reduction of risk of deep vein thrombosis in patients who have had a stroke (CLOTS 3): a multicenter randomized controlled trial. *Lancet* 2013;382:516–524.

5. Dargin J, Medzon R. Emergency department management of the airway in obese adults. *Ann Emerg Med* 2010;56:95–104.
6. Galovic M, Leisi N, Müller M, Weber J, Abela E, Kägi G, Weder B. Lesion location predicts transient and extended risk of aspiration after supratentorial ischemic stroke. *Stroke* 2013;44:2760–2767.
7. Hashiguchi N, Lum L, Romeril E, et al. Hypertonic saline resuscitation: efficacy may require early treatment in severely injured patients. *J Trauma* 2007;62:299–306.
8. Hinchey JA, Shephard T, Furie K, et al. Formal dysphagia screening protocols prevent pneumonia. *Stroke* 2005;36:1972.
9. Hubble MW, Brown L, Wilfong DA, et al. A meta-analysis of prehospital airway control techniques part I: orotracheal and nasotracheal intubation success rates. *Prehosp Emerg Care* 2010;14:377–401.
10. Indredavik B, Rohweder G, Naalsund E, Lydersen S. Medical complications in a comprehensive stroke unit and an early supported discharge service. *Stroke* 2008;39:414.
11. Inouye SK, van Dyck CH, Alessi CA, et al. Clarifying confusion: the confusion assessment method; a new method for detection of delirium. *Ann Intern Med* 1990;113:941.
12. Jones DA, De Vita MA, Bellomo R. Rapid-response teams. *N Engl J Med* 2011;365:139–146.
13. Kamphuisen PW, Agnelli G. What is the optimal pharmacological prophylaxis for the prevention of deep-vein thrombosis and pulmonary embolism in patients with acute ischemic stroke? *Thromb Res* 2007;119:265.
14. Kamran SI, Downey D, Ruff RL. Pneumatic sequential compression reduces the risk of deep vein thrombosis in stroke patients. *Neurology* 1998;50:1683.
15. Karpman C, Keegan MT, Jensen JB, Bauer PR, Brown DR, Afessa B. The impact of rapid response team on outcome of patients transferred from the ward to the ICU: A single-center study. *Crit Care Med.* 2013;41:2284–2291.
16. Kiely DK, Bergmann MA, Murphy KM, et al. Delirium among newly admitted post-acute facility patients: prevalence, symptoms, and severity. *J Gerontol A Biol Sci Med Sci* 2003;58:M441.
17. Langhorne P, Stott DJ, Robertson L, et al. Medical complications after stroke: a multicenter study. *Stroke* 2000;31:1223.
18. Lecky F, Bryden D, Little R, Tong N, Moulton C. Emergency intubation for acutely ill and injured patients. *Cochrane Database Syst Rev* 2008:CD001429.
19. Mace SE. Challenges and advances in intubation: rapid sequence intubation. *Emerg Med Clin North Am* 2008;26:1043–1068.
20. Mann G, Hankey GJ. Initial clinical and demographic predictors of swallowing impairment following acute stroke. *Dysphagia* 2001;16:208.
21. Massey D, Aitken LM, Chaboyer W. Literature review: do rapid response systems reduce the incidence of major adverse events in the deteriorating ward patient? *J Clin Nurs* 2010;19:3260–3273.
22. McCullough GH, Wertz RT, Rosenbek JC. Sensitivity and specificity of clinical/bedside examination signs for detecting aspiration in adults subsequent to stroke. *J Commun Disord* 2001;34:55.
23. McGaughey J, Alderdice F, Fowler R, et al. Outreach and Early Warning Systems (EWS) for the prevention of intensive care admission and death of critically ill adult patients on general hospital wards. *Cochrane Database Syst Rev* 2007:CD005529.
24. Miles A, Zeng IS, McLauchlan H, Huckabee ML. Cough reflex testing in dysphagia following stroke: a randomized controlled trial. *J Clin Med Res* 2013;5:222–233.
25. Murad MH, Stubbs JR, Gandhi MJ, et al. The effect of plasma transfusion on morbidity and mortality: a systematic review and meta-analysis. *Transfusion* 2010;50:1370–1383.
26. Schneider LS, Tariot PN, Dagerman KS, et al. Effectiveness of atypical antipsychotic drugs in patients with Alzheimer's disease. *N Engl J Med* 2006;355:1525.
27. Wijdicks EFM. Neurogenic paradoxical breathing. *J Neurol Neurosurg Psychiatry.* 2013;84:1296.
28. Wong CL, Holroyd-Leduc J, Simel DL, Straus SE. Does this patient have delirium? Value of bedside instruments. *JAMA* 2010;304:779.
29. Younes RN, Aun F, Ching CT, et al. Prognostic factors to predict outcome following the administration of hypertonic/hyperoncotic solution in hypovolemic patients. *Shock* 1997;7:79–83.

2

Fever Control

Body temperature is a critical vital sign, and both high and low values have significance.[34] The simple fact is that sick neurologic patients often become notably febrile during their hospital stay and often early after admission.[19]

Fever is a useful clinical warning sign and may have many infectious and noninfectious causes. In practice, fever is associated with infection in about 50–70% of the cases of acute neurologic injury. Pulmonary infection, tracheal bronchitis, and pneumonia are the most prominent of infectious fevers and exhibit a relationship with the severity of illness. Comatose patients are at higher risk of developing fever from nosocomial pneumonia.

Diagnostic tests should be cost-effective and launching a broad evaluation with every fever spike is nonproductive.[27] Yet, when fever is accompanied by hypotension, patients should be rapidly treated for early sepsis following a comprehensive protocol. Any delay in reversing the situation may cause irreparable secondary brain damage. It is a known clinical observation that untreated high fever with hypotension shock may suddenly and permanently change the neurologic outlook of the patient.

Fever of central origin is particular to patients with acute brain injury.[10,13,16] All the more troubling is that the effects of fever alone are perniciously bad for an acutely injured brain.[4] Evaluation of fever is important, and close control of increasing temperatures could have an impact on outcome (although this is not definitively proven).[2,3,17,35,42] Fever is treated with antipyretic therapy, or cooling, and there is now a better understanding of how to do that effectively. Likewise, the evidence that hypothermia can be therapeutic in any type of brain injury needs to be treated cautiously.

Outside the extremes such as the major neurologic hyperthermia syndromes, there are basically three main questions: How do we respond to a fever spike? How do we best cool down a patient? How quickly should that be done? This chapter provides an overview of the known mechanisms, evaluation of fever, and opportunities for appropriate management.

Principles

There is fever and a febrile response. Fever can be defined and depends on age and possibly also time of the day and acceptable criteria are shown in Table 2.1. The

Table 2.1 **Fever Definition**

Site	Temperature
Oral	Day: t >37.7°C (>100°F)
	Morning: t >37.2°C (>99°F)
	Age >65 y: t >37.8°C (>100°F)
Rectal	t ≥38°C (100.4°F)
	Age > 65y: t>37.2°C (99°F)
Axilla	t≥37.5°C (99.5°F)

febrile response, however, is a more complex manifestation that includes shivering, cutaneous vasoreaction with piloerection, sweating, and most importantly, increased metabolic demands. Excessive temperature elevation, or hyperthermia, is comparatively commonly seen in acute neurologic disorders and must be recognized and adequately treated.

TEMPERATURE FEEDBACKS

How is fever generated? The thermoregulatory center is in the preoptic area (POA) located anterior and rostral to the hypothalamus. One core principle in fever control is that multiple signals can be delivered to this center and the main temperature feeds are the visceral, spinal cord, and brain temperatures.[21,25,26,29] POA can be signaled by an infection that triggers the immune system through so-called pyrogenetic mediators, which may stimulate this center. Any environmental change will be sensed by the skin, and both warm and cool receptors will stimulate the POA and result in a subsequent response.

The responses to a warm and cool environment, and how it is currently understood, are summarized in Figure 2.1.[5,6,45] Briefly, the cutaneous cool and warm receptors activate some of the sensory neurons that innervate neurons in the spinal and trigeminal medullary dorsal horn. These tracts are organized and separated out and, through spinothalamic tracts, connections are made with the somatosensory cortex that helps in signaling. The autonomic response to warmth is sweating and vasodilatation. The autonomic response to cold is vasoconstriction and shivering.

The most problematic clinical issue is when the temperature becomes extremely high, usually defined as a temperature reaching 40°C. This is obviously the result of thermoregulatory failure and is seen in a lesion where the ambient temperature—in combination with dehydration—limits sweating and subsequently results in excessive heat production. This may occur with very unusual clinical syndromes such as malignant hyperthermia or neuroleptic malignant syndrome, but besides neuroleptics there are other drugs that can generate hyperthermia such as atropine, amphetamine, and cocaine. In those situations, hyperthermia apparently results from impaired peripheral heat loss. There is intact regulation, and the normal fever

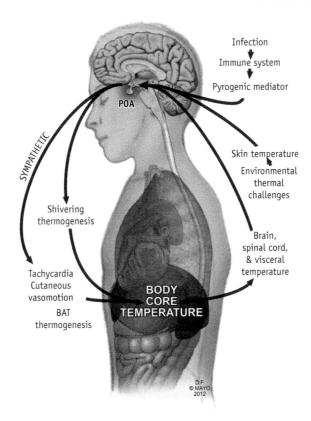

Infection
↓
Immune system
↓
Pyrogenic mediator

POA

SYMPATHETIC

Shivering
thermogenesis

Skin temperature
Environmental
thermal
challenges

Brain,
spinal cord,
& visceral
temperature

Tachycardia
Cutaneous
vasomotion
BAT
thermogenesis

BODY
CORE
TEMPERATURE

D.F.
© MAYO
2012

Figure 2.1 Schematic model of central circuitries underlying autonomic and somatic effector responses for thermoregulation and fever. (adapted from reference 29.)

responses are intact (vasoconstriction and shivering do occur), but the "set point" is elevated. In other words, the heat response mechanism is shifted to a higher value.

Another principle is that fever results in a cardiovascular and metabolic response. Fever causes increased cardiac output that is therefore associated with increased oxygen consumption, carbon dioxide production, and generally increased energy expenditure. Oxygen consumption can increase by approximately 10% per degree Celsius. The metabolic response consists of increased glucocorticosteroid production, increased secretions of growth hormone and aldosterone, but reduced secretion of vasopressin.

FEVER AND THE BRAIN

Increase in brain temperature can worsen prior brain injury.[18] Moreover, it is known that brain temperature is a fraction higher than core body temperature. It has been established that fever not only worsens ischemic injury, but also worsens cerebral edema, increases intracranial pressure, and, in general, confounds

Table 2.2 **Mechanisms Underlying Protective Effects of Hypothermia**

- Prevention of apoptosis
- Reduced mitochondrial dysfunction, improved energy homeostasis
- Reduction of excessive free radical production
- Mitigation of reperfusion injury
- Reduced permeability of the blood-brain barrier and the vascular wall; reduced edema formation
- Reduction of oxygen and glucose requirements
- Depression of the immune response and various potentially harmful proinflammatory reactions
- Anticoagulant effects
- Suppression of epileptic activity and seizures

the general examination of the patient.[24,33,35,37] Markedly febrile patients will have a decreased level of consciousness—or even develop hypoactive delirium—which can rapidly improve with control of fever. Studies in traumatic brain injuries, subarachnoid hemorrhage, stroke, and cardiac arrest have documented that uncontrolled fever is an independent variable of poor outcome.[46]

Fever in itself may have dramatic effect on the brain irrespective of its cause. It may result in increased levels of excitatory amino acids with the end result of free radicals and lactic acid; it may facilitate breakdown of the blood-brain barrier and reduce cytoskeletal stability; and it can eventually lead to cerebral edema, which could impact the degree of brain injury. The most extreme situation is environmental heat stroke. Brain injury often consists of multiple petechial hemorrhages, and the mechanism is not entirely understood. What plays in the mix is rapid fulminant hepatic failure likely due to extreme rhabdomyolysis, with myoglobin plugging small arteries in many organs including the brain. Induced hypothermia could have many protective effects and they are summarized in Table 2.2.

In Practice

The first clinical responsibility is to explain fever and tailor a reasonable workup. The second responsibility is to actively treat fever with a combination of measures. Pharmacological control of fever is notoriously difficult and seldom sustained. Temperature control with cooling devices has markedly improved practice. Sandwiching patients with cooling blankets and ice packs, and even gastric lavage with iced water, is still very effective but slightly more cumbersome. Control of fever is now one of the important additional interventions necessary to control increased intracranial pressure, better manage status epilepticus and to treat hypertensive surges in patients with sympathetic overdrive.

FEVER ASSESSMENT

One way to address the severity of fever is by calculating fever burden. This is defined as a Tmax of 38°C summed from several days. Fever burden is basically a calculation that measures the combined effect of temperature and duration of fever. High fever burden had six-fold increased odds of poor outcome in ischemic stroke and hypothermia may be protective.[20] A high fever burden also may be associated with poor outcome in subarachnoid hemorrhage.[28] Fever burden could be related to the severity of subarachnoid hemorrhage, presence of vasospasm, presence of a ventriculostomy, and a large amount of blood on computed tomography (CT) scan.

The most likely causes of fever are shown in Figure 2.2 and each should be considered.[8,9] Fever, traditionally when defined as fever higher than 38.3°C on several

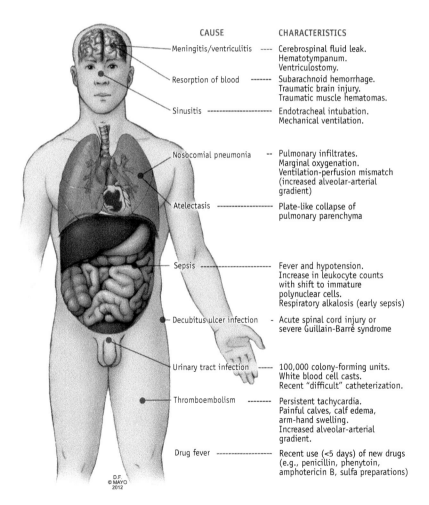

CAUSE | CHARACTERISTICS

Meningitis/ventriculitis ---- Cerebrospinal fluid leak.
Hematotympanum.
Ventriculostomy.

Resorption of blood ------- Subarachnoid hemorrhage.
Traumatic brain injury.
Traumatic muscle hematomas.

Sinusitis ------------------ Endotracheal intubation.
Mechanical ventilation.

Nosocomial pneumonia -- Pulmonary infiltrates.
Marginal oxygenation.
Ventilation-perfusion mismatch
(increased alveolar-arterial
gradient)

Atelectasis ------------------ Plate-like collapse of
pulmonary parenchyma

Sepsis ------------------ Fever and hypotension.
Increase in leukocyte counts
with shift to immature
polynuclear cells.
Respiratory alkalosis (early sepsis)

Decubitus ulcer infection - Acute spinal cord injury or
severe Guillain-Barré syndrome

Urinary tract infection ----- 100,000 colony-forming units.
White blood cell casts.
Recent "difficult" catheterization.

Thromboembolism -------- Persistent tachycardia.
Painful calves, calf edema,
arm-hand swelling.
Increased alveolar-arterial
gradient.

Drug fever ------------------ Recent use (<5 days) of new drugs
(e.g., penicillin, phenytoin,
amphotericin B, sulfa preparations)

D.F.
© MAYO
2012

Figure 2.2 Causes of Fever.

occasions, can be due to not only infections but also malignancy and connective tissue disease that has been undiagnosed. Several laboratory tests may be required for evaluation, including blood cultures, erythrocyte sedimentation rate or C-reactive protein, serum lactate dehydrogenase, the HIV antibody test and viral load, creatinine and phosphokinase, antinuclear antibodies, serum protein electrophoresis, and CT of the abdomen and chest.[22,31] CT of the abdomen may be able to detect a previously undiagnosed abscess or hematoma. CT of the chest may find small nodules that may be indicative of a fungal infection or malignancy. This may lead to bronchoscopy or even mediastinoscopy with mediastinal adenopathy biopsy.

Fever may occur with an invasive procedure or manipulation of an indwelling device.[32] It may also be transiently associated with transfusion of blood products or recently administered drugs. If fever persists, one should expect that at least half of the episodes are of noninfectious origin. Most often it is caused by drug hypersensitivity or "drug fever." Temperature is typically between 39°C and 40°C and may be associated with shaking, chills, and spiking temperatures. Skin rashes may not be present and will make the diagnosis more difficult to establish. Fever is rarely associated with increased white cell counts, but—as expected—peripheral eosinophilia may be seen and erythrocyte sedimentation rate can increase. Often patients with drug-related fever do not have a pulse rate response and are relatively bradycardic. The drugs that possibly cause drug-related fever are antibiotics (particularly the β-lactams), any antiepileptic drug, antiarrhythmics, antihypertensives, diuretics, and even more mundane drugs such as stool softeners. In fact, all of these should be considered when fever occurs after an interval of a week. Antibiotics that less frequently cause drug-related fever are vancomycin, clindamycin, erythromycin, imipenem, quinolones, and aminoglycosides.

Other causes of noninfectious fever that need to be investigated are transfusion reactions, large hematomas at deep body sites, deep venous thrombosis, pulmonary embolus, or any acute hemorrhage. Any patient with intracranial hemorrhage may develop a central cause of fever; this is common in patients after subarachnoid hemorrhage and has been linked to the development of vasospasm (the link between fever and vasospasm may simply be reabsorption of subarachnoid blood). A recent study found central fever in nearly 50% of patients admitted to the neurosciences ICU. Central fever is likely (probability of .90) when cultures are negative, chest X-ray shows no infiltrate, onset of fever is within 3 days of admission and a diagnosis of subarachnoid, intraventricular hemorrhage or brain tumor has been made.[19]

TREATMENT OF FEVER ASSOCIATED WITH BACTEREMIA

The initial approach is to observe and not to respond in a reflexive manner if the patient is hemodynamically stable. If fever persists, all central lines should be removed and cultured.[31,32] In a patient with diarrhea, stool culture and empiric antibiotics can be considered, particularly PRCs against *Clostridium difficile* and vancomycin-resistant *Enterococcus* toxins.

Infectious causes that should be investigated are urinary tract infections, which are mostly nosocomial and may cause bacteremia. Hospital-acquired pneumonia or ventilator-associated pneumonia are the most common causes of infection in seriously ill neurologic patients. Pulmonary infiltrates may not be adequately visualized on chest X ray and chest CT scan may be useful (Chapter 3). Bronchoscopy may be necessary to investigate pulmonary infiltrates, obtain good cultures, and evacuate mucus plugs. Often forgotten are infections caused by sinusitis in a patient who had prior prolonged intubation.[30]

Fever becomes far more problematic if hypotension occurs. Failure to recognize this sign as a manifestation of systemic inflammatory response syndrome (Table 2.3) may lead to a rapidly downward spiraling clinical picture, rapidly crossing the threshold from which improvement is unlikely. These signs should trigger activation of the sepsis-management protocol.[10] The general principles of management of septic shock apply to patients with acute brain injury (Table 2.4).[1,14,38,39] Updated guidelines have been recently published.[12]

Fluid resuscitation should be started emergently with 1,000–2,000 mL of crystalloids over 30 minutes. In patients with acute brain injury, normal saline is preferable to lactated Ringer's solution to avoid fluids with lower tonicity. Colloids (5% albumin) can also be used. The usual target is a mean arterial pressure (MAP) of 65 mm Hg, but a higher target is preferred in patients with low cerebral perfusion values. Serum lactate should be measured quickly and is an important indicator of the seriousness of the situation. A serum lactic acid level greater than 4 mmol/L indicates tissue hypoperfusion and calls for aggressive hemodynamic support. The patient's urinary output needs to be closely monitored for the development of oliguria (less than 20 mL/h).

Norepinephrine is the initial vasopressor of choice. It may be supplemented with low-dose vasopressin (0.03 units per minute) if the blood pressure target is not achieved. Epinephrine and dopamine are reasonable options. However, the pure alpha-adrenergic agonist, phenylephrine, is not a good choice in septic shock because it can reduce cardiac output (i.e., stroke volume) and myocardial dysfunction may accompany sepsis. If the left ventricular ejection fraction is reduced on echocardiogram and shock persists, inotropes such as dobutamine should be started (Table 2.4). After the patient has been successfully resuscitated,

Table 2.3 **Systemic Inflammatory Response Syndrome (SIRS)***

Physiological Variable	Measurement
Body temperature	> 38.5°C or < 35°C
Heart rate	> 90 beats per minute
Respiratory rate	> 20 breaths per minute or $PaCO_2$ < 32 mm Hg
White blood cell count	> 12,000 cells/mm³, 4,000 cells/mm³ or > 10% bands

* SIRS with proven infection defines sepsis. *Source:* Adapted from reference 12.

Table 2.4 **Initial Treatment of Septic Shock with Special Considerations for Neurological Patients**

Start aggressive fluid resuscitation immediately

1–2 L of 0.9% NaCl (may add intermittent infusions of 250 mL of albumin 5%)

Define resuscitation goal

A MAP goal higher than the usual 65 mm Hg may be necessary in neurocritical patients with compromised cerebral perfusion

---

Start vasopressor if MAP below target after fluid challenge

Norepinephrine, low-dose vasopressin, epinephrine

Phenylephrine is not adequate

Obtain echocardiogram and assess systolic function

Start dobutamine if left ventricular ejection fraction is decreased

---

Conservative fluid strategy after resuscitation goal is achieved

Can use diuretics if MAP is stable

Low tidal volume, high PEEP, recruitment manouvers, prone positioning in ARDS

Diagnose the source of infection; start broad-spectrum antibiotics as soon as possible

---

Consider hydrocortisone if vasopressor dependence

Avoid activated human recombinant protein C due to increased risk of ICH

Blood product administration

Consider red blood cell transfusion to keep hemoglobin >9–10 g/dL if cerebral perfusion is compromised

Platelet transfusion to keep platelet count >50,000 if recent ICH or neurosurgery

FFP to correct coagulopathy if recent ICH or neurosurgery

Glucose control

Maintain blood sugars between 140–180 mg/dL

FFP, fresh frozen plasma; ICH, intracranial hemorrhage; MAP, mean arterial pressure. *Source:* From Wijdicks and Rabinstein. *Neurocritical Care.* New York, Oxford University Press, 2012.

fluid administration must be very conservative (i.e., fluid balance even to negative) to prevent complications from fluid overload (principally related to capillary leak leading to pulmonary edema). However, this approach can create a dilemma in certain acute neurological disorders. In patients with brain edema, maintaining a negative fluid balance is actually desirable. Marginal cerebral perfusion pressures (i.e., symptomatic vasospasm) can result in ischemia if there is intravascular volume contraction.

Patients with septic shock not quickly responding to these measures may be treated with corticosteroids (hydrocortisone 50 mg intravenously every 6 hours). Corticosteroids may reduce vasopressor dependency but do not appear to improve survival. In addition, recombinant human-activated protein C must not be administered to patients with intracranial hemorrhage or recent neurosurgery because of the increased risk of hemorrhage.

Early initiation of broad-spectrum antibiotics is crucially important. Ideally, they should be started within the first hour of the diagnosis of septic shock. Pancultures should be obtained before the first antibiotic dose, if at all possible, but cannot delay the start of antibiotics.[11,15]

Septic shock guidelines generally recommend transfusion of red blood cells only when the hemoglobin concentration is below 7 g/dL. However, critically ill neurological patients may have a different target. Improving oxygen-carrying capacity may be particularly beneficial in these patients with compromised cerebral perfusion and recent or persistent hypotension. Transfusion at a higher hemoglobin concentration of 9–10 g/dL should be considered.

HOW TO COOL EFFECTIVELY

The use of cooling devices has significantly improved the management of these patients.[3,14,23,36] Most cooling is achieved with cooling blankets, and many hospitals now have the opportunity to use cooling pads that can keep a stationary temperature. Direct brain cooling is a new area of research and of uncertain benefit. This approach has included nasopharyngeal probes that seem to cool the carotid arteries.[44] Nasal cooling does cool the deep venous sinus at the base of the skull but its effect is questionable.[43] Brain temperature measurement in selected patients may allow monitoring for efficacy but this is not common practice.[40,41]

Rapid cooling can be achieved in controlled hospital settings with well-designed practice protocols, but quick cooling can also be achieved by large-volume (20 mL/kg) cold (refrigerator cold; 4°C) saline, though its effect is short—less than 30 minutes—and may need to be repeated (with 10 mL/kg) until more long-lasting effective measures are available. Intravascular systems may be more efficacious than external cooling devices, but the evidence remains unclear. The current cooling devices can cool the patient rather quickly at a rate of 4°C/h. Most of the cooling devices are able to maintain an adequate set time and overshoots of core temperature have been unusual. A guideline is shown in Table 2.5.

Cooling failure, defined as not reaching a target temperature within 24 hours of starting to lower the core temperature, is variable and usually occurs in 20%–30% of patients. Cooling failure is more common with external cooling and that

Table 2.5 **Therapeutic Hypothermia**

• Control shivering (meperidine or propofol)
• Avoid temperature <30°C
• Aggressively treat infections
• Rewarm (0.2°C–0.5°C per hour)
• Adjust drug levels and increase insulin effect if needed with rewarming

may be an incentive to proceed with endovascular cooling (with its inherent risks of infections and thrombosis). Predisposing factors for cooling failure are high body mass index and early intercurrent infection.

Shivering can be a major complication of fever control, particularly if the temperature overshoots to hypothermia. Shivering is a thermoregulatory response to low ambient temperature; it usually occurs at 35°C and progresses from shivering in the neck musculature to twitching in the thorax and abdomen. If shivering progresses, it may cause gross movements of the upper and lower extremities. Shivering is usually counteracted by opioids. The most effective drugs to control shivering are propofol or meperidine. These drugs have a rapid effect. If these are unsuccessful, clonidine, or a more radically, neuromuscular blocker can be tried. The disadvantage of neuromuscular blockers is that they will mask any seizure activity if it occurs, and patients at high risk of seizures would require continuous EEG monitoring. Moreover, there remains a substantial risk of critical illness neuromyopathy after several days of neuromuscular blockers.

Generally, the best intervention for mild shivering is dexmedetomidine, starting at a dose of 0.2 mcg/kg/h titrating up to 1.5 mcg/kg/h. In addition, propofol 75–100 mcg/kg/min and fentanyl 25 mcg/h or meperidine 100 mg/IM or IV is helpful. Acetaminophen or buspirone are rarely helpful, although in mild cases they may reduce shivering. The dose of acetaminophen is usually 1,000 mg every 4–6 hours and the dose of buspirone 30 mg every 8 hours. It has been empirically found that in some patients, magnesium sulfate 1 mg/h IV aiming at serum magnesium levels of 4 mg can be quite helpful in treating shivering.[7]

"Shivering" may also be a clinical sign in coma.[47] Currently, shivering in comatose survivors of cardiopulmonary resuscitation mostly is observed during hypothermia treatment, but long before the widespread introduction of this treatment modality "shivering" had been reported in the immediate hours and days after anoxic-ischemic injury. The physiologic mechanism in coma is not known, but the shivers—particularly in the absence of piloerection—are likely the result of reticulospinal tract injury.

Putting It All Together

- The five major causes of noninfectious causes of fever are drug fever, blood resorption, deep venous thrombosis (arm and leg), dysautonomia, and major atelectasis
- Temperature control may help in ICP management and secure control
- Temperature control is best achieved with a closed-loop cooling device
- Shivering can be adequately treated with opioids, propofol, dexmedetomidine, or meperidine
- Fever and hypotension should initiate a sepsis management protocol

---

By the Way

- Fever >39.5°C may decrease level of alertness
- Fever after brain injury often has noninfectious causes
- Fever is rarely effectively reduced with drugs
- Fever is a prognostic sign in acute brain injury
- Increased intracranial pressure and seizures may worsen with fever

---

Fever by the Numbers

- ~20% increase in daily water necessity per degree Celsius
- ~10% difference between brain and core temperature
- ~10% increase in cardiac consumption per degree Celsius
- ~5% increase in brain oxygen consumption per degree Celsius
- ~3% difference between axillar and rectal temperature

References

1. American College of Chest Physicians/Society of Critical Care Medicine Consensus Conference: definitions for sepsis and organ failure and guidelines for the use of innovative therapies in sepsis. *Crit Care Med* 1992;20:864–874.
2. Azzimondi G, Bassein L, Nonino F, et al. Fever in acute stroke worsens prognosis: a prospective study. *Stroke* 1995;26:2040–2043.
3. Badjatia N. Hyperthermia and fever control in brain injury. *Crit Care Med* 2009;37:S250–S257.
4. Blatteis CM. Fever: is it beneficial? *Yale J Biol Med* 1986;59:107–116.
5. Boulant JA, Dean JB. Temperature receptors in the central nervous system. *Annu Rev Physiol* 1986;48:639–654.
6. Bratincsák A, Palkovits M. Activation of brain areas in rat following warm and cold ambient exposure. *Neuroscience* 2004;127:385–397.
7. Choi HA, Badjatia N, Mayer SA. Hypothermia for acute brain injury—mechanisms and practical aspects. *Nat Rev Neurol* 2012;8:214–222.
8. Commichau C, Scarmeas N, Mayer SA. Risk factors for fever in the neurologic intensive care unit. *Neurology* 2003;60:837–841.
9. Cunha BA. Fever in the critical care unit. *Crit Care Clin* 1998;14:1–14.
10. Dellinger RP, Schorr C. Severe sepsis in an emergency department: prevalence, rapid identification and appropriate treatment. *Crit Care Med* 2007;35:2461–2462.
11. Cunha BA. Intensive care, not intensive antibiotics. *Heart Lung* 1994;23:361–362.
12. Dellinger RP, Levy MM, Rhodes A. Surviving Sepsis Campaign: international guidelines for management of severe sepsis and septic shock 2012. *Crit Care Med* 2013;41:580–637.
13. Diringer MN, Reaven NL, Funk SE, Uman GC. Elevated body temperature independently contributes to increased length of stay in neurologic intensive care unit patients. *Crit Care Med* 2004;32:1611–1612.
14. Diringer MN; Neurocritical Care Fever Reduction Trial Group. Treatment of fever in the neurologic intensive care unit with a catheter-based heat exchange system. *Crit Care Med* 2004;32:559–564.

15. Eggimann P, Pittet D. Infection control in the ICU. *Chest* 2001;120:2059–2093.
16. Ginsberg MD, Busto R. Combating hyperthermia in acute stroke: a significant clinical concern. *Stroke* 1998;29:529–534.
17. Greer DM, Funk SE, Reaven NL, Ouzounelli M, Uman GC. Impact of fever on outcome in patients with stroke and neurologic injury: a comprehensive meta-analysis. *Stroke* 2008;39:3029–3035.
18. Hickey RW, Kochanek PM, Ferimer H, Alexander HL, Garman RH, Graham SH. Induced hyperthermia exacerbates neurologic neuronal histologic damage after asphyxial cardiac arrest in rats. *Crit Care Med* 2003;31:531–535.
19. Hocker S, Tian L, Li G, et al. Indicators of central fever in the neurologic intensive care unit. *JAMA Neurology* 2014, in press.
20. Kollmar R, Schabitz WR, Heiland S, et al. Neuroprotective effect of delayed moderate hypothermia after focal cerebral ischemia: an MRI study. *Stroke* 2002;33:1899–1904.
21. Kuo FC, Palmer EL, Tseng YH, Doria A, Kolodny GM, Kahn CR. Identification and importance of brown adipose tissue in adult humans. *N Engl J Med* 2009;360:1509–1517.
22. Marik PE. Fever in the ICU. *Chest* 2000;117:855–869.
23. Mayer SA, Kowalski RG, Presciutti M, et al. Clinical trial of a novel surface cooling system for fever control in neurocritical care patients. *Crit Care Med* 2004;32:2508–2515.
24. Mellergard P, Nordstrom CH. Intracerebral temperature in neurosurgical patients. *Neurosurgery* 1991;28:709–713.
25. Morrison SF, Nakamura K, Madden CJ. Central control of thermogenesis in mammals. *Exp Physiol* 2008;93:773–797.
26. Morrison SF, Nakamura K. Central neural pathways for thermoregulation. *Front Biosci* 2011;16:74–104.
27. Mourad O, Palda V, Detsky AS. A comprehensive evidence-based approach to fever of unknown origin. *Arch Intern Med* 2003 10;163:545–551.
28. Naidech AM, Bendok BR, Bernstein RA, et al. Fever burden and functional recovery after subarachnoid hemorrhage. *Neurosurgery* 2008;63:212–217.
29. Nakamura K. Central circuitries for body temperature regulation and fever. *Am J Physiol Regul Integr Comp Physiol* 2011;301:R1207–1228.
30. O'Grady NP, Murray PR, Ames N. Preventing ventilator-associated pneumonia: does the evidence support the practice? *JAMA* 2012;307:2534–2539.
31. O'Grady NP, Barie PS, Bartlett JG, et al. Guidelines for evaluation of new fever in critically ill adult patients: 2008 update from the American College of Critical Care Medicine and the Infectious Diseases Society of America. *Crit Care Med.* 2008;36:1330–1349.
32. O'Grady NP, Alexander M, Burns LA, et al. Summary of recommendations: Guidelines for the Prevention of Intravascular Catheter-related Infections. *Clin Infect Dis* 2011;52:1087–1099.
33. Oliveira-Filho J, Ezzeddine MA, Segal AZ, et al. Fever in subarachnoid hemorrhage: relationship to vasospasm and outcome. *Neurology* 2001;56:1299–1304.
34. Peres Bota D, Lopes Ferreira F, Mélot C, Vincent JL. Body temperature alterations in the critically ill. *Intensive Care Med* 2004;30:811–816.
35. Phipps MS, Desai RA, Wira C, Bravata DM. Epidemiology and outcomes of fever burden among patients with acute ischemic stroke. *Stroke* 2011;42:3357–3362.
36. Polderman KH. Induced hypothermia and fever control for prevention and treatment of neurological injuries. *Lancet* 2008;371:1955–1969.
37. Reaven NL, Lovett JE, Funk SE. Brain injury and fever: hospital length of stay and cost outcomes. *J Intensive Care Med* 2009;24:131–139.
38. Rivers E, Nguyen B, Havstad S, et al; Early Goal-Directed Therapy Collaborative Group. Early goal-directed therapy in the treatment of severe sepsis and septic shock. *N Engl J Med.* 2001;345:1368–1377.
39. Russell JA. Management of sepsis. *N Engl J Med* 2006;355:1699–1713.
40. Schwab S, Schwarz S, Spranger M, Keller E, Bertram M, Hacke W. Moderate hypothermia in the treatment of patients with severe middle cerebral artery infarction. *Stroke* 1998;29:2461–2466.

41. Schwab S, Spranger M, Aschhoff A, Steiner T, Hacke W. Brain temperature monitoring and modulation in patients with severe MCA infarction. *Neurology* 1997;48:762–767.
42. Schwarz S, Hafner K, Aschoff A, Schwab S. Incidence and prognostic significance of fever following intracerebral hemorrhage. *Neurology* 2000;54:354–361.
43. Springborg JB, Springborg KK, Romner B. First clinical experience with intranasal cooling for hyperthermia in brain-injured patients. *Neurocrit Care* 2013;18:400–405.
44. Takeda Y, Hashimoto H, Koji F, et al. Effects of pharyngeal cooling on brain temperature in primates and humans: a study for proof of principle. *Anesthesiology* 2012;117:117–125
45. Virtanen KA, Lidell ME, Orava J, et al. Functional brown adipose tissue in healthy adults. *N Engl J Med* 2009;360:1518–1525.
46. Wang Y, Lim LL, Levi C, Heller RF, Fisher J. Influence of admission body temperature on stroke mortality. *Stroke* 2000;31:404–409.
47. Wijdicks EFM. Shivering in coma. *Arch Neurol* 2009;66:1572.

3

Acute Pulmonary Syndromes

The lungs are often normal in patients before acute brain injury, but ventilation (moving air to lungs) or respiration (exchange of oxygen and carbon dioxide) may become rapidly abnormal in serious and acute neurologic disease. The most common cause of poor ventilation is obstruction when the tongue falls backward into the posterior pharynx. Patients with acute brain injury cannot handle oral secretions very well, and failure to notice such a danger may cause pooling that eventually could lead to bronchial obstruction. Any patient with a decreased level of consciousness—whether brief or prolonged—may have a reduced coughing stimulus. Poor gas exchange may also occur from an abnormal breathing drive. Pulmonary complications are often simply a sign of the times—the ability to aggressively resuscitate and the ability to support severely injured patients. Acute neurologic illness affects lung function through several other possible mechanisms. A supine position changes breathing mechanics, and abdominal breathing, much more than ribcage expansion, now participates in tidal volume generation. The movement of the diaphragm cranially with this body position reduces coughing and reduces functional residual capacity, resulting in pooling secretions and stopping up of alveoli. Mucociliary function decreases simultaneously during immobilization and may cause further injury. Reduced coughing in comatose patients facilitates oropharyngeal colonization, which commonly involves *Streptococcus pneumonia*, *Haemophilus influenzae*, and *Staphylococcus aureus*. Any bedbound patient is at high risk for nosocomial pneumonia, and the microbiology of pathogens may be affected by prior use of antibiotics. In the most severely affected patients with traumatic brain injury or aneurysmal subarachnoid hemorrhage, acute lung injury from rapidly appearing pulmonary edema may evolve into acute respiratory distress syndrome (ARDS).

Although neurogenic pulmonary edema occurs in the more extreme settings, and warrants often prolonged ICU care, elsewhere in the hospital and on the ward other pulmonary disorders are far more frequent. Any physician providing acute care must anticipate the development of atelectasis, pleural effusions, infectious infiltrates, aspiration pneumonitis, and sometimes pulmonary emboli. Aspiration pneumonia due to dysphagia remains a ubiquitous problem.[9,12]

Evaluation of pulmonary problems to a certain extent is part of the medical care of neurologic patients. Respiratory failure leads to hypoxemia and hypercapnia (often both), and therefore is further classified as hypercapnic ($PaCO_2 >$ 50 mm Hg) or hypoxemic ($PaO_2 <$ 50 mm Hg) respiratory failure.

Clinical practice usually pertains to the treatment of pulmonary abnormalities in acute brain injury or in either long-standing or acute neuromuscular disorders. The pertinent questions are: How do we assess and manage abnormal pulmonary function? How do we interpret laboratory values? How do we interpret infiltrates, atelectasis, and pleural effusions on chest X-ray and when is action needed? How do we best prevent pulmonary emboli in immobilized patients? This chapter reviews basic knowledge of pulmonary problems so we can recognize and effectively treat them.

Principles

Respiration is usually a ventilation-perfusion (V/Q) match. A mismatch will occur when perfusion is poor (pulmonary emboli) or lung capillary permeability is poor (pulmonary edema). The pulmonary capillary permeability may also be compromised by migration of activated macrophages in the alveolar space, and this inflammatory reaction may cause damage to type II pneumocytes. The major causes of mismatch are shown in Figure 3.1.

The parts of the lung that do not participate in respiration are known as physiologic dead space, the sum of anatomical and alveolar dead space. The anatomical dead space is the part of the airway system not connected with the alveoli, possibly including the tubing between the Y connector and the patient, the pharynx, and the major conduction airways. The alveolar dead space is the part of the airway system that does not permit gas exchange, in which inspired gas is similar to exhaled gas. This total dead space component of the respiratory system is 20%–30%.

In the alveoli, gases move though diffusion and oxygen is much less diffusible than carbon dioxide (about 20 times less). This is an important physiologic

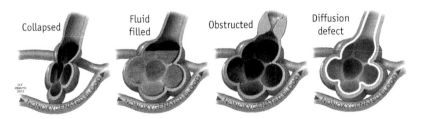

Figure 3.1 Causes of ventilation-perfusion mismatch in acutely ill neurologic patients.

observation because it implies that any process that impairs alveolar diffusion first affects oxygen concentration, leading to hypoxemia. Hypercarbia, because carbon dioxide diffuses so quickly, is only seen when involved areas are large.

One way to do a bedside assessment of gas exchange is the alveolar–arterial oxygen difference (A–a gradient). The alveolar PO_2 (P_AO_2) is calculated using the formula $P_AO_2 = FiO_2 \times 713 - PaCO_2/0.8$. An A–a gradient greater than 20 mm Hg indicates abnormal diffusion or a V/Q defect. Having established that this gradient has increased the FiO_2—usually via inhalation of 100% oxygen (FiO_2 of 1)—we can now determine the degree of mismatch. A significant increase in PaO_2 would indicate a small V/Q mismatch and vice versa.

Another equation helpful in determining the degree of acute lung injury is the PaO_2/FiO_2 ratio: a PaO_2/FiO_2 less than 300 mm Hg (regardless of positive end-expiratory pressure [PEEP]) indicates the beginning of serious respiratory abnormalities. With a PaO_2/FiO_2 less than 200 mm Hg, the patient now has a diagnosis of ARDS.

Drawing blood gases is important because with knowledge of the arterial PaO_2 and arterial PCO_2, pH, and bicarbonate, a good assessment can be made. In a hyperventilating patient, $PaCO_2$ declines and PaO_2 should increase, and the decline and increase are about equal in magnitude. Assuming room air concentration, decrease of $PaCO_2$ by 10 mmHg is associated with PaO_2 rise of 10 mm Hg (strictly speaking slightly less). The $PaCO_2$ can be increased by decreased minute ventilation, increased carbon dioxide production, or increased dead space.

With these parameters two major pulmonary syndromes can be defined: hypercapnic and hypoxemic respiratory failure. Combinations are common. Hypoxemic respiratory failure is usually due to alveolar hypoventilation or V/Q mismatch (or right-to-left shunt). The most common causes are a V/Q mismatch with an abnormal A–a gradient.

Acute hypercapnic respiratory failure is defined by both the A–a gradient and pulmonary function tests. A decreased maximal inspiratory pressure or forced vital capacity identifies an acute neuromuscular disorder. When the respiratory muscles fail, alveolar ventilation is insufficient to eliminate carbon dioxide, and the result is increased tidal volume or respiratory rate. Hypercapnic respiratory failure can be explained as a disconnect between ventilatory supply and ventilatory demand. Alveolar ventilation is inversely proportionate to $PaCO_2$, so with hypoventilation the minute ventilation declines, increasing $PaCO_2$. The hypoxemia seen with hypoventilation is a result of an inadequate ventilatory pump function. Respiratory muscle fatigue in this situation leads to hypercapnia. Hypercapnic respiratory failure is acute if the serum bicarbonate concentration is normal. It is increased in chronic situations because patients with long-standing chronic obstructive pulmonary disease (COPD) and hypercapnia ("the CO_2 retainers")—as a result of renal compensation—have increased serum bicarbonate. Most of the time in hypercapnic respiratory failure there is no hypoxemia—and thus pulse oximeters are useless for monitoring—but hypoxemia may occur if there is no oxygen supplementation. $PaCO_2$ may further increase with oxygen supplementation, which has been explained by removal of the hypoxic drive in a patient with marginal ventilatory drive. The therapy involves oxygen supplementation, but the increase in CO_2 from hypoventilation can only be decreased with mechanical ventilation.

Acute hypercapnia and respiratory acidosis with a normal A–a gradient is commonly due to narcotic or benzodiazepine overdose, which often responds rapidly to antidotes. This situation may also occur with decreased respiratory muscle strength or chest wall abnormalities reducing mechanical function.

Any respiratory rate of more than 30–35 per minute in a patient with extensive X-ray changes indicates an increased ventilatory work load, and a ventilatory assist is needed (biphasic positive airway pressure [BiPAP] or endotracheal intubation and full mechanical ventilation). Once mechanical ventilation has been initiated, hypercapnia and respiratory acidosis can be artificially corrected. This can be accomplished by increasing minute ventilation ("blowing off CO_2") and increasing PEEP to open up collapsed alveoli. Increasing diuresis is another way to reduce pulmonary edema.

In Practice

The most common clinical disorders in acute neurologic disorders associated with acute hypoxemic respiratory failure and V/Q mismatch are atelectasis or large lung field collapse, aspiration pneumonitis, pulmonary embolism, and pulmonary edema (cardiac or neurogenic). The clinical features of acute hypoxemia are fairly consistent and include restlessness, tachypnea, tachycardia, and, sometimes, hypertension and peripheral vasoconstriction.

Management decisions are often determined by bedside chest X-ray. Despite the potential for a long list of possibilities, most abnormalities seen in acutely ill neurologic patients are a major pulmonary collapse, pleural effusion, pneumonia, pulmonary edema, and just simply fluid overload. One can expect these abnormalities in any patient who has become suddenly dyspneic and tachypneic. Examples of common chest X-ray abnormalities are shown in Figure 3.2.[8]

The chest X-ray is also carefully viewed for placement of the endotracheal (ET) tube, which should be 3–5 cm from the carina, half the distance between the medial ends of the clavicle and carina. (carina can be found at T5-T7 level.) The ET tube has a tendency to slide through the right main bronchus due to a shallow angle. In addition, the ET tube position can change 2–4 cm with flexion of the neck and therefore should be several centimeters above the carina.[20]

Acute atelectasis is basically an airless part of the lung created by resorption after obstruction (excessive secretions, mucus plug or even aspiration of a foreign body) or compression (pleural fluid, air, or blood with mass effect). Atelectasis is

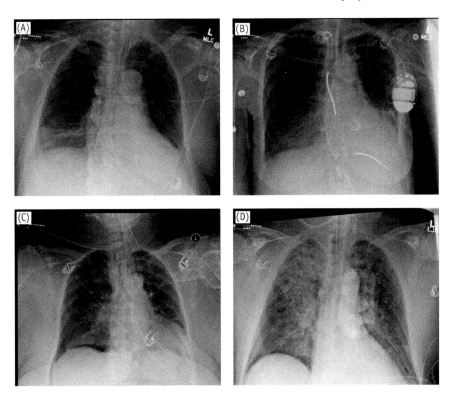

Figure 3.2 X-ray examples of pleural and pulmonary abnormalities. A: Right lower lobe plate atelectasis. B: left pleural effusion. C: right pneumothorax. D: Diffuse (neurogenic) pulmonary edema.

commonly seen in elderly patients, obese patients, and prior smokers, all of which are at higher risk after any sort of immobilization.[1] Usually the lung collapses at the most dependent regions, thus consolidations are seen in the lower lobe.[5] The left lower lobe is most frequently affected by atelectasis. It may initially be seen as a subsegmental plate-like configuration. When a lobe atelectasis occurs, opacity is seen, resulting in volume loss. This presents itself as a disappearance of the diaphragm, air bronchograms, and usually a large field of increased density. Computed tomography (CT) scan of the chest may show these abnormalities in finer detail. A significant improvement is usually seen after a bronchoscopy is performed to suck out the bronchial secretions. In some patients thoracocentesis is needed.[3]

A fluid overload pattern is frequently seen in acutely ill neurologic patients. These chest opacities may have been related to aggressive fluid resuscitation and may be an overshoot in poorly hydrated patients, patients treated with fresh frozen plasma, and in drug-induced hypotension. (A typical example is a patient who has been intravenously loaded with fosphenytoin treated with several boluses of fluid to overcome the hypotension.) The radiographs usually show the development of pleural effusions.

Infection is more difficult to diagnose on X-ray of the chest. Radiographs should be evaluated for segmental infiltrate, pleural effusion, hilar enlargement, and new air space shadows and air bronchograms.[13,14,19] CT scan may be necessary to diagnose empyema or the development of a pulmonary abscess. Healthcare-acquired pneumonia (HAP) or ventilator-associated pneumonia (VAP) is increasingly due to multidrug-resistant or extremely drug-resistant pathogens.[2] These include *Pseudomonas aeruginosa*, *Acinetobacter* species, *Klebsiella pneumonia*, and carbapenems containing *Enterobacteriaceae* (Chapter 9). Pneumonia is usually treated with a β-lactam and a macrolide using 7-day treatment. *S. pneumonia* remains the most common cause of community-acquired pneumonia.

The use of oral gastric decontamination in combination with parenteral antibiotics is often considered, but there is a great likelihood this will lead to more antibiotic resistance in the intensive care unit. A recent meta-analysis found that the effectiveness of subglottic suctioning for the prevention of VAP is associated with reduction in the incidence of VAP and duration of mechanical ventilation.[16] It is a simple technique that can reduce the aspiration of contaminated secretions. Oral care with tooth brushing did not impact on risk of ventilator associated pneumonia.[1] New methods are to use a silver-coated ET tube that can prevent VAP by eluding silver into the environment, where it acts as a bactericidal agent.[11]

Aspiration is a significant risk factor for pneumonia, particularly in the elderly. Aspiration pneumonia may be a cause of admission in 10% (age >80 years) and may not necessarily be related to a neurologic cause of aspiration. This may be related to age-associated changes in oropharyngeal and gastroesophageal motility that promote aspiration into the bronchi. Aspiration needs to be further investigated with video fluoroscopy; if there is no evidence of spilling over in the bronchi, then often only thin liquids, nectar, or honey-thickened liquids are allowed.

Another important clinical fact is that pulmonary infections and respiratory compromise from pneumonia are more common in patients with COPD. Mechanical ventilation also increases the risk of mortality in patients with COPD. COPD is often associated with a history of smoking and also increases the risk of sepsis and ARDS.[5,6,7,15] In these patients there is not only higher risk but also higher incidence of *Pseudomonas aeruginosa*.[4,17] Premorbid COPD associated with advanced age, severe respiratory disease, and cardiovascular or renal organ dysfunction all increase mortality.[22]

Pleural effusions develop frequently in hospitalized patients and also quite frequently in acutely ill neurologic patients. Mostly it becomes apparent on a chest X-ray and will show blunting or disappearance of a costophrenic angle—it can occur with as little as 100 mL of fluid and sometimes it appears as if the diaphragm is elevated (the so-called veiling effect). The pleural effusion does cause atelectasis and eventually poor alveolar transport, shunting, and hypoxemia. However, it may go both ways. Atelectasis causes a decrease in pleural pressure and allows transudate into the pleural space. Larger pleural effusions then cause atelectasis from pressure.

Pleural effusions are also found in patients with anasarca (marked hypo-albuminemia), in patients with pneumonia progressing into an empyema, and in patients with chronic renal failure. Pleural effusions are mostly transudate and may improve with improvement of atelectasis and thus PEEP—transiently increasing to 15 cm water. If this is not helpful and oxygen supplementation remains high (FiO_2 more than 0.7), a thoracocentesis may be considered.

The decision to treat pulmonary infiltrates is obviously difficult. Empirical use of antibiotics in order to avoid missing an infection is common, and there is no good alternative. In most patients, a broad spectrum of empirical treatment is initiated and starts with a third-generation cephalosporin with an aminoglycoside, but a third- or fourth-generation cephalosporin alone may be sufficient, avoiding the toxicity of many of the aminoglycosides. Cefepime may be preferred in *P. aeruginosa*. The broad-spectrum quinolones can be very useful, largely because they penetrate well into secretions. Vancomycin is the preferred drug if *S. aureus* pneumonia is suspected. Dosing of vancomycin should be carefully monitored. (vancomycin dose of more than 4 grams a day increases nephrotoxicity.) The treatment of anaerobic pneumonias is best initiated with the use of ertapenem, but this drug slightly reduces the seizure threshold and should be avoided in patients at high risk of seizures (Chapter 9).

The most concerning pulmonary condition is a pulmonary embolus, and many neurologists have learned over the years to consider this potentially fatal illness in any patient with sudden respiratory distress.[21] However, the clinical presentation of pulmonary embolism is rarely dramatic in acutely ill neurologic patients and often far more subtle, with unexplained mild tachycardia, brief oxygen desaturations, and unexplained fever while chest X-ray remains normal. Moreover, up to 10% of patients with pulmonary emboli will maintain normal oxygenation. Massive main bronchial artery or saddle pulmonary embolism may cause sudden cardiovascular collapse, but this is unusual and not commonly diagnosed intra vitam. Albeit very nonspecific, a new-onset cardiac arrhythmia should in any immobilized patient raise the suspicion of a pulmonary embolus.

The clinical features of pulmonary embolism thus have a low specificity. Approximately 60% have tachypnea or tachycardia, 10% have right heart failure with hypotension, 1% have acute left heart failure with hypotension, and one in three patients is asymptomatic. A blood gas will show reduced $PaCO_2$ and PaO_2 and an increased A–a gradient. Electrocardiographic changes are nonspecific but could show a deep S wave in lead I and a deep Q wave in lead III. (This S1Q3 sign is not common).

Computed tomographic angiogram of the chest is commonly performed and is highly specific. CT scans may not detect subsegmental emboli if there are infiltrates or large areas of atelectasis preventing good scrutiny of the basal lung fields.

Treatment of pulmonary embolism depends on the size of the embolus and where it came from. Emboli are usually from deep vein thrombosis in leg veins but when central lines have been placed—or are still in situ—thrombi may have reached the subclavian vein. Patients with massive pulmonary embolus are usually in shock from acute cor pulmonale, which justifies aggressive treatment with thrombolytic agents. Thrombolytic agents improve hemodynamic variables, but do not change mortality rates. In these circumstances, tissue plasminogen activator—0.6 mg/kg over 15 minutes—can be administered. This is a major quandary because administration of thrombolytics may substantially increase the probability of hemorrhage in a recent hemispheric infarct, cause enlargement of an existing cerebral hematoma, cause hemorrhage in a prior brain tumor, or cause bleeding in a neurosurgical operating bed. As a last resort, emergency embolectomy or extracorporeal membrane oxygenation may be indicated in patients with no improvement in hemodynamic measurements.

Supportive treatment therefore remains the mainstay of management in patients with pulmonary emboli. Correcting hypoxemia with higher FiO_2 of 0.6–1.0 is effective. Patients with low cardiac output are best served by inotropes in an attempt to improve right ventricular performance. Volume expansion in patients in shock from massive pulmonary embolization is indicated only for those who need additional volume to counter the effects of positive-pressure ventilation. Fluid loading may cause further right-ventricular distension and more ventricular strain. High-intensity anticoagulation (activated partial thromboplastin time level between 60 and 90) is started with a 40–80 unit/kg intravenous push loading of intravenous heparin followed by 25,000 units/250 mL at 100 units per mL (18 units/kg) infusion. Administration of warfarin can begin 48 hours after the start of heparinization. Retrievable filter devices should be placed in patients with an absolute contraindication to anticoagulation and in patients with recurrent episodes despite adequate anticoagulation.

Acute lung injury can lead to increased lung water. The accumulation of pulmonary edema can be from increased permeability, with flux of protein solute increasing oncotic pressure and increasing alveoli flooding. Acute injury to the brain or brainstem may cause massive ("flash") pulmonary edema. Conditions that have been associated with neurogenic pulmonary edema are ganglionic hemorrhage, aneurysmal subarachnoid hemorrhage, primary brainstem hemorrhage, status epilepticus, and penetrating brain injury. The clinical picture is very specific, almost always appearing soon after the initial brain injury. The clinical entity may be mistaken for other pulmonary conditions, such as massive aspiration pneumonia or pulmonary contusion. Management of neurogenic pulmonary edema focuses on recruitment of collapsed alveoli with PEEP to correct the marked V/Q mismatch. Mechanical ventilation with PEEP nearly always reverses the condition, and radiographic improvement is evident within hours. Ventilation in a prone position can significantly improve oxygenation. In most severe cases, extracorporeal membrane oxygenation has been advocated with variable success. If the origin of pulmonary edema is not clear or it could be due to stress cardiomyopathy, echocardiogram is warranted, and if poor ventricular function is confirmed, dobutamine (5–15 μg/kg/min) to improve ventricular forward flow could be considered.

Respiratory muscle function in mechanically ventilated patients commonly is impaired and may have to do with ventilator settings (overassistance or underassistance).[4] There may be other acute pulmonary or respiratory problems in patients recently placed on ventilators, making the ventilatory support seem inadequate. Several complications of endotracheal intubation have been described. Most often there is right mainstem intubation. This is a consequence of a natural tendency to further insert the tube after placement seems secure, probing the tube further into the right mainstem. This may be immediately noted after auscultation, and misplacement is easily found on X-ray if checked after placement.

There are important initial clinical signs to look for in a mechanically ventilated patient with acute respiratory distress and a sudden increase in respiratory rate. Agitated patients with an acute central nervous system catastrophe have an increased respiratory drive culminating in large minute volumes asynchronous with the mechanical ventilator. In other mechanically ventilated patients, breathing suddenly could change to tachypnea or complete arrhythmic breathing.

A best approach is to first disconnect the patient from the ventilator and provide manual bagging with large tidal volumes and 100% oxygen. Immediate clinical improvement with 100% oxygen points toward a ventilator-related cause, which may simply indicate inappropriate ventilator settings. For example, a patient on continuous positive airway pressure, or CPAP, may become drowsy and hypoventilate, and will breathe much better with volume-assisted breaths. Leaks in the connections are not uncommon and should be identified.

However, if the pulse oximeter does not indicate immediate improvement in oxygenation, the next step is to check the patency of the airway and to listen carefully. Usually such a condition involves accumulated secretions, in which case deep tracheal suctioning must be performed. If asymmetrical breath sounds are heard on auscultation of the lungs, mainstem intubation or obstruction may be present. Asymmetrical breath sounds are not specific. Many conditions can produce these findings, including acute pneumothorax and pleural effusions. Failure to resolve respiratory distress after an attempt at tracheobronchial suctioning is followed by emergency chest X-ray to determine the position of the tube and an attempt to diagnose a primary pulmonary problem (pneumothorax, pulmonary edema) or abdominal distension (gastric distension, bowel perforation). Fiberoptic bronchoscopy may follow in patients with diminished breath sounds to clear excess secretions.

A much less common pulmonary problem is acute pneumothorax. This may occur with central line placement or trauma to the chest, and can be associated with a therapeutic bronchoscopy, a procedure that has dramatically increased in use over the recent years. Another cause is a right pneumothorax, which occurs when (particularly after a right mainstem intubation) the bronchus is suddenly exposed to a large positive-pressure breath. Another suspicious contributing factor is recent use of large tidal volumes (>12 mL/kg) and high PEEP values (>15 mm Hg).

Acute pneumothorax is probable in patients who have unilateral absence of breath sounds and certainly when there is additional sudden hypotension. In a mechanically ventilated patient, most pneumothorax could be diagnosed clinically and can be confirmed on X-ray. In some patients pneumothorax may develop quickly and a tube thoracostomy should be placed immediately.

By the Way

- Acute hyperventilation and hypoxemia may be a pulmonary embolus
- Unexplained fever may be due to subsegmental pulmonary emboli
- Some patients have COPD and will benefit from bronchodilators
- A–a gradient calculation is dependent on FiO_2 manipulation
- Antibiotic coverage must be broad early but should be narrowed
- Aspiration is mostly self-limiting, and antibiotics may not be needed

---

Acute Pulmonary Syndromes by the Numbers

- ~95% of pulmonary emboli are from leg deep venous thrombosis
- ~95% of inferior vena cava filters remain patent
- ~60% of patients in neurologic intensive care unit develop pleural disease
- ~30% of bronchoalveolar lavage reveals specific organisms
- ~25% of nosocomial infections in the intensive care unit are pulmonary
- ~10% of aspiration is related to intoxication

Putting It All Together

- Many patients with acute neurologic injury start with normal lung function
- Atelectasis and pleural effusions are common concerns
- Acute bronchial mucus plug is another common concern
- Reduce time on the ventilator to reduce chance for ventilator-associated pneumonias
- Consider pulmonary emboli if chest X-ray does not fit with clinical picture.

References

1. Alhazzani W, Smith O, Muscedere J, Medd J, Cook D. Toothbrushing for critically ill mechanically ventilated patients: a systematic review and meta-analysis of randomized trials evaluating ventilator-associated pneumonia. *Crit Care Med* 2013;41:646–655.
2. Carratalà J, Garcia-Vidal C. What is healthcare-associated pneumonia and how is it managed? *Curr Opin Infect Dis* 2008;21:168–173.
3. Collins TR, Sahn SA. Thoracocentesis: clinical value, complications, technical problems, and patient experience. *Chest* 1987;91:817–822.
4. Doorduin J, van Hees HW, van der Hoeven JG, Heunks LM. Monitoring of the respiratory muscles in the critically ill. *Am J Respir Crit Care Med* 2013;187:20–27.
5. Esper AM, Martin GS. The impact of comorbid conditions on critical illness. *Crit Care Med* 2011;39:2728–2735.
6. Fernández-Sabé N, Carratalà J, Rosón B, et al. Community-acquired pneumonia in very elderly patients: causative organisms, clinical characteristics, and outcomes. *Medicine (Baltimore)* 2003;82:159–169.
7. Fowler AA, Hamman RF, Good JT, et al. Adult respiratory distress syndrome: risk with common predispositions. *Ann Intern Med* 1983;98:593–597.
8. Henschke CI, Yankelevitz DF, Wand A, Davis SD, Shiau M. Accuracy and efficacy of chest radiography in the intensive care unit. *Radiol Clin North Am* 1996;34:21–31.
9. Kikuchi R, Watabe N, Konno T, et al. High incidence of silent aspiration in elderly patients with community-acquired pneumonia. *Am J Respir Crit Care Med* 1994;150:251–253.
10. Kollef MH. Hospital-acquired pneumonia/ventilator-associated pneumonia prevention: truth or dare! *Crit Care Med* 2011;39:2015–2016.
11. Lorente L, Blot S, Rello J. New issues and controversies in the prevention of ventilator-associated pneumonia. *Am J Respir Crit Care Med* 2010;182:870–876.
12. Marik PE, Kaplan D. Aspiration pneumonia and dysphagia in the elderly. *Chest* 2003;124:328–336.
13. Milne ENC, Pistolesi M, Miniati M, Giuntini C. The radiologic distinction of cardiogenic and noncardiogenic edema. *AJR* 1985;144:879–894.
14. Milne ENC, Pistolesi M. *Reading the Chest Film: A Physiologic Approach.* St. Louis (MO), Mosby Year Book, 1993.
15. Montgomery AB, Stager MA, Carrico CJ, Hudson LD. Causes of mortality in patients with the adult respiratory distress syndrome. *Am Rev Respir Dis* 1985;132:485–489.
16. Muscedere J, Rewa O, McKechnie K, et al. Subglottic secretion drainage for the prevention of ventilator-associated pneumonia: a systematic review and meta-analysis. *Crit Care Med* 2011;39:1985–1991.
17. Rello J, Rodriguez A, Torres A, et al. Implications of COPD in patients admitted to the intensive care unit by community-acquired pneumonia. *Eur Respir J* 2006;27:1210–1216.

18. Nyquist P, Stevens RD, Mirski MA. Neurologic injury and mechanical ventilation. *Neurocrit Care* 2008;9:400–408.

19. Ruskin JA, Gurney JW, Thorsen MK, Goodman LR. Detection of pleural effusions on supine chest radiographs. *AJR* 1987;148:681–683.

20. Underwood GH, Newell JD. Pulmonary radiology in the intensive care unit. *Med Clin North Am* 1983;67:1305–1324.

21. Wijdicks EFM, Scott JP. Pulmonary embolism associated with acute stroke. *Mayo Clin Proc* 1997;72:297–300.

22. Wildman MJ, Sanderson CF, Groves J, et al. Survival and quality of life for patients with COPD or asthma admitted to intensive care in a UK multicentre cohort: the COPD and Asthma Outcome Study (CAOS). *Thorax* 2009;64:128–132.

4

Acute Cardiac Syndromes

Cardiac injury has been acknowledged as a consequence of acute brain injury and often is associated with clinical manifestations. The observation that electrocardiographic (EKG) abnormalities and even brief cardiac arrhythmias are common soon after the ictus may not necessarily cause concern. In fact, for many cardiologists the question of whether these changes either are typically fitting with the neurologic injury or signal a greater problem is not really a question—the changes are usually benign.[1] Arrhythmias may arise from certain regions in the brain, including the insular cortex, cingulate cortex, and the amygdala, but the connection is not so clear in clinical practice, where there is often more widespread or multifocal hemispheric involvement (see volume *Recognizing Brain Injury*).[17,30]

The problem in part is that one should not accept that cardiac manifestations with acute brain injury are a minimal risk. Brief tachyarrhythmias causing demand ischemia—leading to serum troponin leak—are likely underrecognized. This may occur in previously healthy patients but is more likely in patients with prior (known or, more likely, previously unknown) coronary or myocardial disease.[2,36]

The question of whether the patient with acute brain injury is developing a cardiac syndrome is highly pertinent and urgent. The presentation usually includes new EKG changes, and these abnormalities could closely resemble acute ST-segment myocardial infarction (STEMI) or non-STEMI. In other patients, there are new cardiac arrhythmias such as supraventricular and ventricular ectopy, tachycardia, and atrial fibrillation.

Underlying heart failure or coronary syndrome is common in patients who are admitted after an ischemic stroke.[5] Obesity, in itself, increases the risk of coronary artery disease and sleep apnea with or without pulmonary hypertension, deep vein thrombosis, and pulmonary emboli, all of which are more prevalent. Any patient with a history of ischemic heart disease, prior stroke, history of decompensated heart failure or prior heart failure, diabetes mellitus, or renal insufficiency may warrant further assessment, certainly if a major endovascular procedure under anesthesia or a surgical procedure is anticipated.[3] Conditions that require intensive care management are: unstable coronary syndromes, including unstable or severe angina or a prior myocardial infarction; decompensated heart failure, supraventricular arrhythmias with a ventricular rate of >100 beats/min, symptomatic bradycardia, and newly recognized ventricular tachyarrhythmia. Any heart valve disease that includes severe aortic stenosis or symptomatic mitral stenosis also places the patient at increased risk during any procedure that may include surgery.

There are unique challenges when it comes to cardiac complications. How much is really within the provenance of an attending neurologist? When is a cardiologist urgently needed for advice? What can be expected in certain acute neurologic disorders, and which patients need more close monitoring? This involves a basic assessment but also recognition of acute coronary syndromes, treatment of acute atrial fibrillation, and evaluation for a temporary pacemaker. Full justice cannot be granted to this topic here, but this chapter highlights the most commonly encountered problems and frequent cardiac management concerns in acutely ill neurologic patients.

Principles

The first core principle is a comprehensive cardiac evaluation. Any physician should obtain a simple set of data that could classify the patient in a certain risk category. This includes a full "bare essentials" cardiac examination. History of unstable angina is important but likely not readily available or known. Cardiac auscultation may yield important findings. Specific attention should be directed toward new regurgitation murmurs, abnormal heart rhythms, and abnormal cardiac heaving or thrusting. Most patients with uncomplicated STEMI or non-STEMI have a normal blood pressure. With emerging cardiogenic shock and when systolic blood pressure declines below 90 mm Hg, the skin may become cool and clammy—due to global decrease in cerebral perfusion patients become disoriented and confused. The heart rate may increase or decrease, often depending on whether left ventricular failure is emerging. Respiratory rate is normal in most acute cardiac manifestations, but periodic breathing may signal the appearance of cardiac failure.

Auscultation of the heart is a specialized skill that only experienced cardiologists have, but there are simple observations that can be useful. Generally the clinical finding with the highest accuracy for predicting heart failure is a third heart sound. Appearance of a third sound (gallop rhythm) indicates left ventricular dysfunction—all best heard at the apex with a left recumbent turn of the patient—and a result of increased filling pressure of the left ventricle. Diffuse wheezing and rales are also signs of profound left ventricular failure. The cardiac evaluation is summarized in Table 4.1.

Table 4.1 **Cardiac Evaluation**

• Cardiac auscultation for murmurs
• Gallop rhythm
• Crackles
• Apex displaced
• Edema
• Tachycardia >100/min.
• Jugular venous distension

A second core principle is to assess the patient's volume status. Is there volume overload or low cardiac output? Jugular venous pressure may be increased or normal in patients with heart failure and is not a useful test if not examined with assessment of the hepatojugular reflux (compression of the right upper quadrant for one minute with persistent rise of the jugular venous pressure after release). Its presence is highly indicative of increased cardiac filling pressures. Pulsus alternans (strong beat followed by a weak beat) is diagnostic of a low-output state, but most patients are also cool, dry, have facial pallor, and may have peripheral cyanosis.

A third core principle in early evaluation of a patient with a possible cardiac syndrome is to specifically look for high-risk electrocardiograms, those that predict serious cardiac arrhythmias. An admission electrocardiogram should be carefully scrutinized for the presence of Q waves, significant ST elevation or depression (deviation of 0.5 mm or more), increased QT interval, or a new bundle branch block. Any of these abnormalities should be explained and possible causes identified.

A fourth core principle is to know how and why to obtain more specific tests. This includes serum cardiac troponin and B-type natriuretic peptide (BNP). Cardiac troponins are proteins that control the calcium-mediated interaction between actin and myosin. The troponin complex consists of troponin C, which binds calcium; troponin I, which binds actin-myosin interactions, and troponin T, which attaches to the troponin complex by binding to tropomyosin and improves contraction. BNP is elevated in congestive heart failure. Of greater importance, a normal BNP virtually excludes heart failure and is useful if the diagnosis is uncertain.

If there is a serious evolving situation patients will need a bedside echocardiogram. This study provides information regarding left and right ventricular failure, ejection fraction, chamber size, regional wall motion, and estimation of right ventricular pressure to anticipate pending pulmonary hypertension. The presence of a thrombus, pericardial effusion, valvular dysfunction, or valvular strands is an important piece of information.

In Practice

There are several clinical dilemmas that come up frequently. Many decisions are made on an ad hoc basis and may often early involve a cardiologist's opinion. Further details can be found in the volume Recognizing Acute Brain Injury.

APPROACH TO MYOCARDIAL ISCHEMIA

Serum troponin can be used to exclude ("rule out") myocardial infarction or diagnose ("rule in") myocardial infarction. Common sense, however, dictates that it takes multiple parameters to diagnose myocardial infarction.[7,11] One important lesson is not to get too intimidated by elevations of serum troponin in acutely ill neurologic patients.[9,12,13,16] Troponin leaks do indicate myocardial injury and can be a result of any acute brain injury with hypertension causing acute ventricular strain.[27,28] However, in itself, an isolated elevation of troponin level does not indicate an acute coronary syndrome. The significance of cardiac troponin increase is a commonly asked question. The serum cardiac troponin level in normal individuals is considered to lie within the range of 0.1–0.2 ng/L, and this is due to normal myocyte loss.[31,35] The sensitivity of troponin T measurements has significantly improved, and this high-sensitivity of cardiac troponin I and T may cause difficulties with its interpretation. Usually cardiac troponin can be detected about 2 hours after onset of myocardial injury, but if the clinical suspicion is high, blood samples will have to be redrawn 3–6 hours later. Cardiac troponin levels can remain elevated up to 7 days for troponin I and 2 weeks for troponin T. Generally, peak troponin T indicates infarct size and is a reliable predictor of left ventricular function at 3 months and major adverse effects at 1 year.[26] Elevated troponin T is also predictive of 30-day mortality in a patient with acute myocardial ischemia. But, if by 6 hours after the onset of symptoms the troponin is not elevated, the chance of a myocardial infarction is very low.

For neurologists, it is important to know that most patients with stress cardiomyopathy have only a modest rise in cardiac troponin that peaks within 24 hours. The magnitude of increase in cardiac troponin is much less than that measured in STEMI, and there is also a less steep rise. Troponin T, more than 0.6 ng/mL, or troponin I, more than 0.5 ng/mL does not fit with neurogenic stress cardiomyopathy.[31] There are also many nonthrombotic causes of increased cardiac troponin, including demand ischemia in patients with supraventricular tachycardia or during atrial fibrillation with rapid ventricular response, significant anemia, hypotension, or hypovolemia. Cardiac troponin may also be increased by direct myocardial damage from contusion or chest trauma; and can be seen as a result of myocarditis, prior chemotherapy, direct-current cardioversion, or cardiac surgery. Pulmonary emboli or pulmonary hypertension may cause myocardiac strain and result in elevated troponin. Chronic (or acute on chronic) renal failure and sepsis are also well-known causes of an elevated cardiac troponin.[11] Generally, increase in troponin can be seen in stable angina where the numbers are approximately 0.01 mcg/L. A small myocardial infarction or myocarditis or pulmonary emboli is typically in the 1 mcg/L range. A large territorial myocardial infarction is between 10 and 100 mcg/L.

Cardiac troponin has been found increased after every acute brain injury, but all studies have reported random values with wide intervals between measurement and ictus and no consistent correlations with outcome. Cardiac troponin can increase after any type of ischemic or hemorrhagic stroke and has been related to prognosis.[22,24] Mostly the prevalence varies between 0% and 35% and contractile dysfunction and EKG changes such as ST depression and ST-wave inversion are also seen in these patients. Patients with increased troponin levels after an acute stroke additionally often have features of myocardial ischemia on EKG and a greater risk of mortality than patients who do not have a troponin rise.[14,15]

In general, a measurement of cardiac troponin within the first hour after presentation with evidence of a change (Δ) within first hours, coupled with the clinical picture and abnormal echocardiogram, and certainly if troponin levels are sufficiently high, should warrant cardiologic consultation and appropriate medical therapy.

APPROACH TO STRESS CARDIOMYOPATHY

Stress cardiomyopathy may present with "flash" pulmonary edema and relative hypotension progressing to severe hypotension. In these instances neurogenic pulmonary edema is often wrongly diagnosed, and cardiac failure is not considered. For most physicians more common considerations in acute cardiac failure, are acute systolic or diastolic dysfunction, acute valvular dysfunction, new cardiac arrhythmia, acute myocardial infarction, and free wall rupture or pericardial tamponade. Sepsis or long-standing cardiovascular surgery and prolonged cardiopulmonary bypass are other causes. Stress cardiomyopathy is common after a brain injury but often is not considered. Conditions predisposed to it are aneurysmal subarachnoid hemorrhage (SAH), status epilepticus and posterior reversible encephalopathy syndrome (PRES).

The diagnosis of stress cardiomyopathy is based on several criteria: (1) a major acute unexpected stressful event or acute brain injury; (2) transient left ventricular wall motion abnormalities involving the apical or midventricular myocardial segments but with wall motion abnormalities extending beyond the single epicardial coronary distribution; (3) absence of obstructive coronary artery disease or angiographic evidence of acute plaque rupture that could be responsible for the observable wall motion abnormality; and (4) new EKG abnormalities such as transient ST elevation or diffuse T-wave inversion or troponin elevations (Table 4.2).[4] Clinical management includes consideration of early treatment with β-blockers, but also inotropes. The treatment of stress cardiomyopathy is largely determined by its presentation.[18-20,38] Usually, patients have a decreased ventricular function

Table 4.2 **Diagnostic Criteria Proposed by Mayo Clinic for Apical Ballooning Syndrome**

- Transient hypokinesis, akinesis, or dyskinesis of the left ventricular midsegments with or without apical involvement. Regional wall motion abnormalities extend beyond a single epicardial vascular distribution.

- Absence of obstructive coronary artery disease or angiographic evidence of acute plaque rupture.

- New EKG abnormalities (ST-segment elevation or T-wave inversion) or modest elevation in cardiac troponin.

- Absence of:
  - pheochromocytoma
  - myocarditis

Source: From reference 4.

but are not in shock. In these patients, close observation, avoidance of fluid overload, and cardiac rhythm control, if needed, is sufficient, and the abnormalities will reverse.

If shock occurs, patients need to be treated immediately and aggressively. If the patient has developed acute heart failure with congestion, intravenous vasodilators are used with diuretics. Vasodilators, however, cannot be used if there is symptomatic hypotension. In patients with cardiogenic shock, defined as significant hypotension of systolic blood pressure <90 mm Hg due to impaired contractility, high intracardiac filling pressures, and marked tissue hyperperfusion, intravenous inotropes should be administered acutely. Mostly dopamine is administered at a dose of 5–20 mcg/kg/min. Dopamine increases contractility and heart rate through activation of the β-adrenergic receptors and also mediates vasoconstriction through the activation of α-receptors in the periphery.[32,33] A much less attractive option is IV norepinephrine, which increases afterload without significantly increasing cardiac output.

In certain circumstances, dopamine and milrinone (a phosphodiesterase inhibitor) can significantly increase cardiac output through peripheral vasodilatation and reduction in cardiac afterload. Milrinone reduces right and left ventricular filling pressures but also mean arterial pressure. Therefore, there is a risk of hypotension with milrinone; moreover, the drug also has a long half-life, making it a somewhat complicated drug in this setting. In extreme instances, a severe stress cardiomyopathy with hypotension has been treated with an intraaortic balloon counterpulsation pump (IABP).[25] These balloon pumps are based on counterpulsation, where blood pumped or displaced is synchronized with the normal cardiac cycle. It augments the diastolic pressure and reduces systolic pressure. It reduces left ventricular afterload and left ventricular wall tension and, through that, diminishes the oxygen demand. This will eventually lead to higher mean arterial pressures.

Another presentation of acute cardiac failure syndrome is severe hypertension with pulmonary congestion. Many of these patients have good left ventricular function but poor diastolic function, which results in acute pulmonary edema due to increased pulmonary capillary wedge pressure. Systolic heart failure is often associated with renal failure and a result of marked hypoperfusion. Worsening renal failure leads to fluid retention and worsening cardiac failure. Continuous renal replacement therapy allows both control of intravascular volume and correction of electrolytes.

To summarize, management of stress cardiomyopathy may involve hemodynamic augmentation, but exposing patients to a sympathetic pressor agent such as phenylephrine or norepinephrine to combat hypotensive effects should be considered counterintuitive given that catecholamine toxicity is likely a mechanism contributing to the original cardiac damage. Therefore these patients are better treated with inotropic medications such as dopamine or other inotropic agents such as milrinone. The mainstay of treatment of acute cardiac failure remains adequate oxygenation (may require noninvasive ventilation or endotracheal intubation), pain control with IV morphine, diuretics, and blood pressure control. Treatment of acute cardiac failure with pulmonary edema requires aggressive diuresis with IV furosemide but not exceeding 100 mg in the first 6 hours. Replacement of potassium and magnesium is needed. Vasodilators (sodium nitroprusside and nitrates) are only administered in patients with hypertensive type of congestive heart failure and have been controversial due to their potential for hypotension (and decrease in coronary perfusion) and reflex tachycardia. Inotropic support with dopamine or dobutamine and milrinone (in refractory cases) is needed in some patients, but vasopressors and vasopressin can be considered. Intraaortic balloon pump counterpulsation or extracorporeal membrane oxygenation are last-resort options.[21,34]

It is also often pertinent to improve fluid overload and congestion with loop diuretics such as furosemide infusion of 1 to 5 mg/h. Higher doses of furosemide may be needed but should not exceed 20 mg/h because of a considerable risk of permanent deafness from furosemide-induced cochlear damage. It also requires frequent electrolyte measurements and supplementation. Intravenous vasodilators such as nitroprusside decrease preload and afterload but can only be used if there is no evidence of hypotension or risk of hypotension. It also has been established that angiotensin-converting-enzyme (ACE) inhibitors cannot be used in these patients until at a later stage when the patient is more stabilized. It is equally important not to start or increase β-blockade in cases of decompensated heart failure.

APPROACH TO AN ACUTE CORONARY SYNDROME

The major proportion of acute coronary syndromes is non-STEMI in about 2/3 of all myocardial infarctions.[10] STEMI is a life-threatening clinical syndrome that—in neurologic patients—may not be associated with chest pain or pressure but

Table 4.3 **American College of Cardiology/American Heart Association ST-Segment Elevation Myocardial Infarction (STEMI) Diagnosis Guidelines**

• ST-segment elevation ≥1 mm (0.1 mV) in 2 or more adjacent limb leads
• ST-segment elevation ≥1 mm (0.1 mV) in precordial leads V4 through V6
• ST-segment elevation ≥2 mm (0.2 mV) in precordial leads V1 through V3
• New left bundle-branch block

Source: From reference 3.

may manifest itself with shortness of breath, nausea, and vomiting in comatose patients with acute brain injury. Many EKG changes falsely suggest STEMI and turn out to be transient repolarization disturbances not related to myocardial injury. Patients with coronary artery disease who develop an acute brain injury, however, may have an acute or partial occlusion of the coronary artery as a result of activation of the sympathetic nervous system resulting in catecholamine circulation.

STEMI criteria are well defined by the American College of Cardiology and the American Heart Association (Table 4.3).[3] After the diagnosis is established by EKG, troponin, echocardiography, or coronary angiogram, the therapy of acute coronary syndromes is reasonably well established and all patients should immediately receive 325 mg of chewable aspirin (Figure 4.1). Aspirin reduces mortality by 25% and blocks β-activation by limiting thromboxane production via the cyclooxygenase pathway.[20] Current guidelines recommend against the routine use of β-blockers for acute STEMI. The administration of β-blockers to patients with acute coronary syndromes may lead to increased incidence of cardiogenic shock and may nullify the reduction of recurrent ischemia and reinfarction following reperfusion therapy.[6,8,37] It is important to rapidly establish whether the patient is a candidate for revascularization either through administration of fibrinolytic therapy or primary percutaneous coronary intervention. In patients with acute neurologic disease, fibrinolytic therapy is often contraindicated because of the presence of an intracranial hemorrhage, recent ischemic stroke, recent traumatic brain injury, or even the presence of a brain tumor. The common presence of hypertension, with a diastolic blood pressure >100 mm Hg, in patients with acute brain injury is also a relative contraindication. Therefore, it is imperative in these patients to provide immediate reperfusion therapy and percutaneous coronary intervention (PCI) in a cardiac catheterization laboratory.[23,29,33] PCI may be problematic in acute brain injury (recent cerebral hemorrhage, large territorial cerebral infarction, hemorrhagic contusions, ventriculostomy in situ, and so forth) given the need for anticoagulation or dual antiplatelet agents to maintain stent patency.

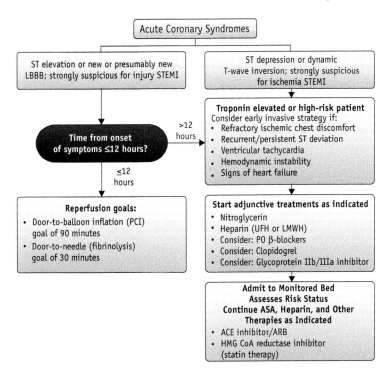

Figure 4.1 Acute coronary syndromes algorithm. (Adapted from reference 26.)

APPROACH TO TACHYARRHYTHMIA

Cardiac arrhythmias are usually innocuous after acute neurologic illness but become concerning if patients have developed myocardial injury or have preexisting morbidity. A first important check is to see whether common causes for cardiac arrhythmias have been excluded. These are: drugs prolonging QTc interval (often haloperidol and atypical antipsychotics), antiepileptic drugs in high doses, therapeutic hypothermia or other cooling intervention, high doses of propofol, and displacement of a central catheter in the atrium. These are all correctable causes. The three most common tachyarrhythmias that are seen in a acutely ill neurologic patient are sinus tachycardia, supraventricular tachycardia and atrial fibrillation with rapid ventricular response (Figure 4.2). Sinus tachycardia is most common and mostly due to dehydration and a compensatory response to hypotension. It may be pain or agitation too. Fluid bolus are usually helpful and rate improves. Supraventricular tachycardia is often due to illness and improves with carotid massage or adenosine followed by metoprolol.

Sinus tachycardia

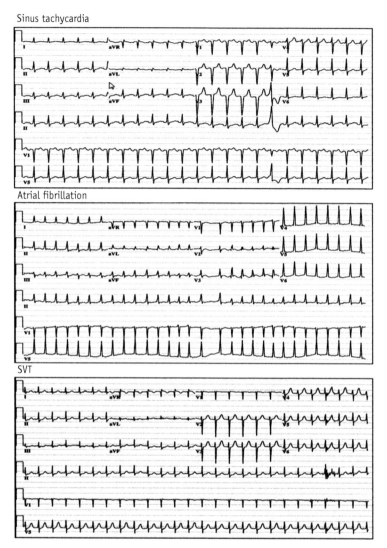

Figure 4.2 Three tachyarrhythmias: Sinus tachycardia, atrial fibrillation and rapid ventricular response and supraventricular (narrow complex) tachyarrhythmia (SVT).

Atrial fibrillation with a subsequent development of rapid ventricular response is a quite common occurrence after acute brain injury.[38] In some instances it may have been facilitated by discontinuation of medication to allow "permissive hypertension." The main principle is to control the rapid ventricular rate, particularly if it results in a hemodynamic unstable arrhythmia. The approach is usually to slow the ventricular rate with either a β-blocker or a calcium channel blocker. Digoxin has a slow onset of action and therefore is not useful in acute treatment. Digoxin,

Table 4.4 **Recommendations for Temporary Transvenous Pacing**

• Asystoles
• Symptomatic bradycardia (includes sinus bradycardia with hypotension and type I second-degree AV block with hypotension not responsive to atropine)
• Bilateral BBB (alternating BBB, or RBBB with alternating LAFB/LPFB)
• New or indeterminate age bifascicular block (RBBB with LAFB or LPFB, or LBBB)
• Mobitz type II second-degree AV block

however is a very useful long-term agent and should not be easily dismissed as treatment. Acute control of atrial fibrillation with rapid ventricular response can be attained with the use of metoprolol given as an intravenous bolus of 5 mg slowly over 2 minutes. (It may be repeated every 5 minutes to a total dose of 15 mg.) An alternative approach is to use an esmolol bolus of 5 mg/kg followed by an infusion starting at 100 mcg/kg/min and increasing to 200 mcg/kg/min. Calcium channel blockers have become most frequently used, and diltiazem given via intravenous bolus of 0.25 mg/kg followed by an infusion of 5–15 mg/h often will control the ventricular rate within a matter of minutes. Direct-current cardioversion may be indicated in unstable patients or those refractory to medical therapy.

Bradycardias are commonly seen in acute brain injury and may have no consequences if the patient remains asymptomatic. It is a common occurrence in patients with a new mass, acute hydrocephalus, crowded posterior fossa due to tumor, and in the setting of dysautonomia in acute neuromuscular disease. Symptomatic bradycardia (usually syncope with hypotension) is an indication for temporary pacing. It may particularly be needed if the patient has a reversible condition such as antiarrhythmic drug therapy overdose, or in the setting of acute myocardial infarction. IV atropine usually suffices, but if it reoccurs pacing may be needed. Indications for pacing are in Table 4.4.

Cardiac arrhymias requires complete evaluation and this book cannot address management of cardiac arrhythmias in detail. Initial management of commonly seen arrhythmias is shown in Table 4.5.

APPROACH TO PREOPERATIVE RISK ASSESSMENT

Older patients with preexisting medical conditions are at risk of postoperative cardiac complications. This risk is already increased in patients with two or more "cardiac medications" (β-blockers, diuretics, calcium channel blockers, ACE inhibitors, and any antiarrhythmic drugs). Common postoperative complications are atrial fibrillation with rapid ventricular rate and acute non-STEMI.

A detailed review of the perioperative cardiac risks and guidelines has been published by the American Heart Association. A procedure such as a craniotomy is

Table 4.5 **Guidance for the treatment of common Cardiac Arrhytmias**

Arrhythmia	Therapy
Sinus tachycardia	Fluids, esmolol
Sinus bradycardia	Atropine, cardiac pacing
Atrial fibrillation	Diltiazem, esmolol, amiodarone
Multifocal atrial tachycardia	Verapamil or metoprolol
Junctional rhythm	Atropine
Atrioventricular block	Cardiac pacing
Ventricular tachycardia	Cardioversion
Torsades de pointes	Magnesium sulfate

Adapted from Wijdicks EFM. The Practice of Emergency and Critical Care Neurology, Oxford University Press, New York, 2010.

at intermediate surgical risk with a reported cardiac arrest and nonfatal myocardial infarction rate of less than 5%. However, cardiac complications are up to five times more common in emergency neurosurgical procedures. Generally, the risk of perioperative myocardial infarction in patients with no evidence of coronary disease (defined by EKG, history of angina, or coronary angiogram) is low.

The risk of cardiac complications increases significantly in patients with unstable coronary syndromes, decompensated congestive heart failure, arrhythmias, and severe valvular disease. A full cardiologic evaluation, if time allows, is needed.

Putting It All Together

- In acute neurologic disease brief troponin rise without EKG changes may indicate insignificant myocardial injury

---

By the Way

- Acute bradycardias occur with acute mass effect, any large hemispheric stroke, or acute dysautonomia and seldom need pacing
- Discontinuation of β-blockade for "permissive hypertension" in acute ischemic stroke may lead to tachycardia and demand ischemia
- Vasodilator therapy way be needed in acute heart failure and hypertension
- Dopamine and/or norepinephrine when cardiogenic shock is present
- Acute aneurysmal rupture may present with unconsciousness and "acute coronary syndrome" but coronary angiogram is often unrevealing

---

Acute cardiac syndromes by the Numbers

- ~70% of patients with SAH have repolarization abnormalities
- ~60% of patients with fatal status epilepticus have myocardial injury
- ~60% of patients with SDH have serious cardiac arrhythmias
- ~30% of comatose patients with SAH may have stress cardiomyopathy
- ~20% of brain dead patients have cardiac dysfunction preventing organ donation

---

- Stress cardiomyopathy may require aggressive treatment for cardiac shock with dopamine and milrinone
- STEMI may require immediate revascularization because fibrinolysis is often contraindicated in patients with acute brain injury
- New onset atrial fibrillation with rapid ventricular response is a common cardiac arrhythmia after acute brain injury and very responsive to β blockade or diltiazem
- Craniotomy has a low risk of perioperative myocardial infarction

References

1. Agarwal S, Lyon A, Nachev P, Everitt A. The nervous heart: a case report and discussion of an under-recognized clinical problem. *QJM* 2009;102:807–809.
2. Amarenco P, Steg PG. Stroke is a coronary heart disease risk equivalent: implications for future clinical trials in secondary stroke prevention. *Eur Heart J* 2008;29:1605.
3. Anderson JL, Adams CD, Antman EM, et al. 2012 ACCF/AHA focused update incorporated into the ACCF/AHA 2007 guidelines for the management of patients with unstable angina/non-ST-elevation myocardial infarction: a report of the American College of Cardiology Foundation/American Heart Association Task Force on Practice Guidelines. *J Am Coll Cardiol* 2013;61:e179–e347.
4. Bybee KA, Prasad A. Stress-related cardiomyopathy syndromes. *Circulation* 2008;118: 397–409.
5. Chin PL, Kaminski J, Rout M. Myocardial infarction coincident with cerebrovascular accidents in the elderly. *Age Ageing* 1977;6:29.
6. Ellis SG, Tendera M, de Belder MA, et al. Facilitated PCI in patients with ST-elevation myocardial infarction. *N Engl J Med* 2008;358:2205–2217.
7. Fure B, Bruun Wyller T, Thommessen B. Electrocardiographic and troponin T changes in acute ischaemic stroke. *J Intern Med* 2006;259:592–597.
8. Fuster V. Fine-tuning therapy for acute coronary syndromes. *N Engl J Med* 2010;363:976–977.
9. Garrett MC, Komotar RJ, Starke RM, et al. Elevated troponin levels are predictive of mortality in surgical intracerebral hemorrhage patients. *Neurocrit Care* 2010;12:199–203.
10. Giugliano RP, Braunwald E. The year in non-ST-segment elevation acute coronary syndrome. *J Am Coll Cardiol* 2009;54:1544–1555.

11. Haaf P, Drexler B, Reichlin T, et al. High sensitivity cardiac troponin in the distinction of acute myocardial infarction from acute cardiac non-coronary artery disease. *Circulation* 2012;126:31–40.

12. Hays A, Diringer MN. Elevated troponin levels are associated with higher mortality following intracerebral hemorrhage. *Neurology* 2006;66:1330–1334.

13. Jensen JK, Atar D, Mickley H. Mechanism of troponin elevations in patients with acute ischemic stroke. *Am J Cardiol* 2007;99:867.

14. Jensen JK, Kristensen SR, Bak S, et al. Frequency and significance of troponin T elevation in acute ischemic stroke. *Am J Cardiol* 2007;99:108–112.

15. Kerr G, Ray G, Wu O, Stott DJ, Langhorne P. Elevated troponin after stroke: a systematic review. *Cerebrovasc Dis* 2009;28:220–226.

16. Kumar S, Selim MH, Caplan LR. Medical complications after stroke. *Lancet Neurol* 2010;9:105.

17. Laowattana S, Zeger SL, Lima JA, et al. Left insular stroke is associated with adverse cardiac outcome. *Neurology* 2006;66:477.

18. Lazaridis C, Pradilla G, Nyquist PA, Tamargo RJ. Intra-aortic balloon pump counterpulsation in the setting of subarachnoid hemorrhage, cerebral vasospasm, and neurogenic stress cardiomyopathy. Case report and review of the literature. *Neurocrit Care* 2010;13:101–108.

19. Lee VH, Connolly HM, Fulgham JR, et al. Tako-tsubo cardiomyopathy in aneurysmal subarachnoid hemorrhage: an underappreciated ventricular dysfunction. *J Neurosurg* 2006;105:264–270.

20. Libby P. Mechanisms of acute coronary syndromes and their implications for therapy. *N Engl J Med* 2013;368:2004–2013.

21. Macrea LM, Tramèr MR, Walder B. Spontaneous subarachnoid hemorrhage and serious cardiopulmonary dysfunction—a systematic review. *Resuscitation* 2005;65:139–148.

22. Maramattom BV, Manno EM, Fulgham JR, et al. Clinical importance of cardiac troponin release and cardiac abnormalities in patients with supratentorial cerebral hemorrhages. *Mayo Clin Proc* 2006;81:192.

23. McKay RG, Dada MR, Mather JF, et al. Comparison of outcomes and safety of "facilitated" versus primary percutaneous coronary intervention in patients with ST-segment elevation myocardial infarction. *Am J Cardiol* 2009;103:316–321.

24. Naidech AM, Kreiter KT, Janjua N, et al. Cardiac troponin elevation, cardiovascular morbidity, and outcome after subarachnoid hemorrhage. *Circulation* 2005;112:2851–2856.

25. Nussbaum ES, Sebring LA, Ganz WF, Madison MT. Intra-aortic balloon counterpulsation augments cerebral blood flow in the patient with cerebral vasospasm: a xenon-enhanced computed tomography study. *Neurosurgery* 1998;42:206–213.

26. O'Connor RE, Brady W, Brooks SC, et al. Part 10: acute coronary syndromes: 2010 American Heart Association Guidelines for Cardiopulmonary Resuscitation and Emergency Cardiovascular Care. *Circulation* 2010;122:S787–S817.

27. Parekh N, Venkatesh B, Cross D, et al. Cardiac troponin I predicts myocardial dysfunction in aneurysmal subarachnoid hemorrhage. *J Am Coll Cardiol* 2000;36:1328–1335.

28. Prosser J, MacGregor L, Lees KR, et al. Predictors of early cardiac morbidity and mortality after ischemic stroke. *Stroke* 2007;38:2295.

29. Riezebos RK, Tijssen JG, Verheugt FW, Laarman GJ. Percutaneous coronary intervention for non ST-elevation acute coronary syndromes: which, when and how? *Am J Cardiol* 2011;107:509–515.

30. Samuels MA. The brain-heart connection. *Circulation* 2007;116:77–84.

31. Sharkey SW, Lesser JR, Menon M, et al. Spectrum and significance of electrocardiographic patterns, troponin levels, and thrombolysis in myocardial infarction frame count in patients with stress (tako-tsubo) cardiomyopathy and comparison to those in patients with ST-elevation anterior wall myocardial infarction. *Am J Cardiol* 2008;101:1723–1728.

32. Thomas SS, Nohria A. Hemodynamic classifications of acute heart failure and their clinical application: an update. *Circ J* 2012;76:278–286.

33. Trost JC, Lange RA. Treatment of acute coronary syndrome: Part 1: Non-ST-segment acute coronary syndrome. *Crit Care Med* 2011;39:2346–2353.
34. Tung P, Kopelnik A, Banki N, et al. Predictors of neurocardiogenic injury after subarachnoid hemorrhage. *Stroke* 2004;35:548–551.
35. Twerenbold R, Jaffe A, Reichlin T, Reiter M, Mueller C. High-sensitive troponin T measurements: what do we gain and what are the challenges? *Eur Heart J* 2012;33:579–586.
36. Vingerhoets F, Bogousslavsky J, Regli F, Van Melle G. Atrial fibrillation after acute stroke. *Stroke* 1993;24:26–30.
37. Wong CK, White HD. Medical treatment for acute coronary syndromes. *Curr Opin Cardiol* 2000;15:441–462.
38. Yoshimura S, Toyoda K, Ohara T, et al. Takotsubo cardiomyopathy in acute ischemic stroke. *Ann Neurol* 2008;64:547–554.

5

Nutrition Assessment

Delivery of adequate calories to patients with acute neurologic disease, most of whom are able to tolerate enteral feeding presents some challenges but is relatively easy most of the time. Parenteral feeding is rarely needed—only in patients who have developed adynamic ileus as a result of opioids, barbiturates, or simply long-term immobilization. Parenteral nutrition—despite availability of a premixed infusate—complicates monitoring and management of the patient and increases the risks of infectious complications due to central line placement and more intensive control of hyperglycemia.

What are the issues to consider with nutrition? First, as a matter of fact, patients with an acute brain injury or acute progressive neuromuscular disease do have abnormal swallowing mechanisms, which makes it difficult to safely feed them orally. Swallowing difficulties are not easily noted, and the severity of it all is often misjudged. Dysphagia becomes clear during feeding, and there are still patients in the hospital who unnecessarily aspirate, followed by a rapidly developing pneumonitis. Second, it has been well appreciated that the more severely ill will benefit from early feeding.[1,2,10,25] In other words, postponing enteral feeding may lead to worsening of the clinical condition, particularly in patients who already had inadequate food intake before admission. Third, deficiencies in nutrition may be present unknowingly. For example, patients with advanced amyotrophic lateral sclerosis may be diagnosed only after significant weight loss and may present not only with respiratory failure but also severe ketoacidosis. Fourth, any patient with acute neurologic illness most likely also has a catabolism that exceeds anabolism and would need to have nutritional support to meet the body's demands. Just placement of a nasogastric tube followed by a standard nutrition formula may temporize the issue initially, but long-term considerations are necessary.

There are multiple nutrition guidelines for sick and critically ill patients—these are A.S.P.E.N., ESPEN, SCCM, and CCCPG guidelines.[14,15,17,18,20,21,27,28] As expected, adherence to guidelines is variable due to lack of sufficient evidence in many of the guidelines, but many surmise that (1) early enteral feeding is necessary, (2) enteral feeding is superior to parenteral feeding,[36] and (3) some supplements may be beneficial in some critically ill patients (i.e., fish oils, supplemental anti-oxidants, and glutamine).[4,5,7,16,26,30] Very little is known regarding the usefulness of direct calorimetry when compared with calculation using known equations, the use of prokinetics, the use of arginine, and if probiotics are useful.[37,38,39] In fact, the caloric and amino acid/protein target is virtually unknown in acutely ill and critically ill neurologic patients. Overfeeding leads to hyperglycemia, hyper-triglyceridemia, and other negative effects.[5] Insulin resistance is commonly seen in critically ill patients. Hyperglycemia has been found to be one of the most important determinants of complications and even prognosis.

When it comes to nutritional support of the patient, any physician has to make decisions soon after admission and, in the process of doing so, answer two crucial questions: Can I feed the patient and how should I feed the patient?[32] In this chapter, the core principles of nutrition in an acutely ill neurologic patient and its practical problems are discussed. (The impact of acute brain injury on the gastrointestinal function is discussed in the volume Recognizing Brain Injury.) Nutrition not only provides energy to the patient, it may also modulate an inflammatory state, improve immunocompetence, and impact on pharmacological administration.

Principles

One of the first core principles is to approach the nutritional needs of the patient in a more comprehensive way. Patients can tolerate extended periods of semistarvation because—expectedly—the body responds to decreased energy intake by reduction of the basal metabolic rate and favors a state in which the fat supplies are used as primary fuel. The metabolic rate in a patient with a neurocatastrophe is increased (hypermetabolism), and rather than depletion of fat, protein stores from lean body mass are rapidly mobilized.[8,21] The major physiologic changes as a result of increased metabolic rate are fever, leukocytosis, hyperglycemia, hypoalbuminemia, and increased blood urea nitrogen. Moreover, many alterations in trace element homeostasis may be due to the acute phase response.

Some other basic principles should be discussed. The patient's comorbidities should be recognized. It is important to know whether the patient has preexisting liver or renal dysfunction, whether additional attention to glycemic control is needed, and what part nutrition will provide in the total fluid intake. It is usually immediately obvious, but physicians should have a sense of the degree of malnutrition. Severe protein energy malnutrition and multiple micronutrient deficiencies are very common in sick patients but also in chronic alcoholics or drug addicts. Malnutrition is also common in the elderly and in nursing home patients. Chronic pulmonary obstructive disease is associated with a significantly lower body mass index (BMI)—and general frailty—and nutrition here is also is difficult to manage. Thus, another core principle is to supplement where needed.

The most important vitamin to consider is thiamine (vitamin B1), because several well-defined syndromes are associated with its deficiency. Thiamine exists in muscle stores (and in a very small percentage in erythrocytes as thiamine pyrophosphate) and is an absolutely necessary cofactor in the Krebs and glycolytic cycles involved in carbohydrate metabolism. Because thiamine is a cofactor for transketolase, a deficiency is reflected by reduced erythrocyte transketolase levels. A diet rich in glucose—most notably a rapid intravenous infusion of glucose—leads to thiamine deficiency and may eventually produce metabolic (lactic) acidosis. Chronic malnutrition, sepsis, burns, and long-term parenteral nutrition are major factors, as well as patients with acute renal failure being treated with continuous renal replacement therapy. Because brain thiamine is low in the first place, it is a vulnerable site.[24] Wernicke-Korsakoff syndrome can be recognized by a confusional state, horizontal or vertical nystagmus, gaze palsy, and ataxia of gait. The dose of thiamine in an established Wernicke-Korsakoff syndrome is much higher and should be 300 mg IV for 3 days and oral absorption should be considered insufficient or frankly poor. Thiamine IM (50–100 mg) must be administered for several more days to prevent more signs (complete ophthalmoparesis and stupor) in severely thiamine-deficient patients. Magnesium (1 g IM as undiluted 50% solution) acts as a cofactor for transketolase activity and may have to be administered in addition.

A third core principle is to determine the energy requirements (Table 5.1). This is a weight-based calculation using 20–40 kcal/kg/day, or using equations such as the Harris-Benedict equations.[34] After caloric requirements are known, the protein requirements are calculated; normally protein is provided using 1.2–1.75 g/kg/day. In patients with excessive protein loss, for example, patients with severe diarrhea, the requirements can be increased to 2 g/kg/day.

It is well known that the lowest mortality initially is associated with obese patients, but the BMI has a U-shaped association with mortality.[11] The risk of mortality may already be increased in the patient with a normal BMI between 18 and 25 kg/m². The most problematic issue is how to predict the energy requirement in an obese person.[19,35] Using actual body weight will overestimate caloric needs because adipose tissue is less metabolically active. Usually an adjusted weight with a 25% stress factor is used, or the patient receives 21 kcal/kg actual weight. Hypocaloric feeding with at least 2 g/kg ideal body weight per day of protein is the best approach for nutrition support that will prevent complications of overfeeding such as hyperglycemia and fluid retention. Protein requirement in obese patients is based on ideal body weight (IBW), with a goal of 2 g/kg/IBW/day for a BMI of 30–40 and 2.5 g/kg/day for a BMI of >40. After feeding is started, a goal should be set that should be at least 60% of calorie requirements.

Table 5.1 **Estimated Energy Requirements**

Calories:	
BMI <30: Use 25–30 kcal/kg ABW/day _____ kcal	
BMI >30: Use 11–14 kcal/kg ABW/day _____ kcal	
Protein:	
BMI <30: Use 1.2–2.0 g protein/kg ABW/day _____ g protein	
BMI 30–40: Use >2.0 g protein/kg IBW/day _____ g protein	
BMI >40: Use 2.5 g protein/kg IBW/day _____ g protein	

ABW = actual body weight; IBW = ideal body weight. (From reference 20 used with permission.)

The nutrient formulas are divided into specialty formulas and formulas that have additional pharmaconutrients. Provision of trace minerals such as selenium, zinc, manganese, and copper is important, particularly in patients with infectious disease. Administration of vitamin C, vitamin E, and selenium for several days seems to improve length of stay and reduce mortality.[6]

There are several "specialty" formulas tailored toward patients with chronic organ failure. Specialty formulas include pulmonary formulas that have a high lipid content, which will decrease carbon dioxide production. Hepatic failure formulations are usually supplemented with branched-chain amino acids that reduce the protein content and might be useful in patients who have hepatic failure treated with lactulose.[12] Renal failure formulations also are markedly reduced in total protein and somewhat reduced in phosphorous and potassium. A typical enteral nutrition formula is isotonic to serum. It provides a caloric density of 1 kg/mL and includes essential vitamins, minerals, and micronutrients.

In Practice

The aspiration risk may be high despite precautions. These are: sips of water between meals, providing thick liquid foods, sitting upright during meals, minimize talking during meals, small bites, empty mouth before adding more. Thus enteral nutrition is the preferred route of feeding in any acutely ill or critically ill patient, including acutely ill neurologic patients.[14,16] It is recommended to start nutrition within the first 24 to 48 hours after admission.[9] This may seem obvious, but when hospitals are audited it is noted that this rarely occurs in ICU settings. A combination of enteral and parenteral nutrition may be tried, but rarely for more than a few days to a week and mostly in overtly malnourished patients or patients who can absolutely not tolerate enteral feeding. The enteral route remains the preferred practice because parenteral nutrition is associated with higher cost and higher risk.

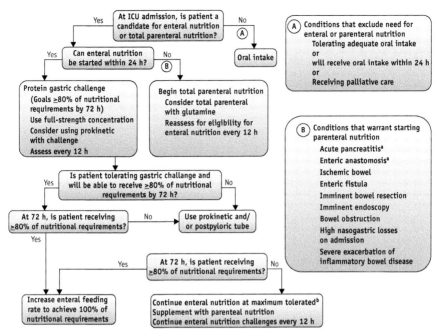

Figure 5.1 Evidence-based feeding guideline. (Adapted from reference 9.)

[a]May still opt for elemental formulation
[b]Clinical indications of enteral feeding intolerance induce clinically significant diarrhea, readily apparent abdominal distension, increased abdominal girth, clinically detected aspiration or gastric residuals >200 mL for nasogastric feeds

The caloric intake continues to be a major determinant of future nutrition status. Functional lean body mass will decline rapidly if nutrition is insufficient, and nutrition will restore the balance between protein breakdown and protein synthesis. Unfortunately, the most common reason for poor nutritional intake is multiple procedures that result in interruption of nutritional intake or insufficient attention by the attending physician.[34] Observational studies have also found that the energy intake is low, with a mean of approximately 1,000 kcal/day in mechanically ventilated patients—this would correspond to 13 kcal/kg in an 80-kg patient and this is significant underfeeding.

Figure 5.1 shows an algorithm on how to start enteral nutrition based on the A.S.P.E.N. guidelines.[14] Enteral nutrition should not be delayed when there are clear signs of intestinal motility such as bowel sounds, flatus, and stools. Gastric residual volume, stool frequency, presence of diarrhea, and bowel sounds are important during continuous assessment.

In the vast majority of patients with acute neurologic disease, feeding is through a nasogastric feeding tube—often also to avoid aspiration when signs are not so clear. The nasogastric feeding tube is typically placed without difficulty; however, its adequate placement can be checked on a simple abdominal X-ray image. The

Table 5.2 **Ten Pointers for Interpreting an X-Ray Image to Check for Correct Placement of Nasogastric Tube**

• Can you see the tube?
• Does the tube path follow the esophagus?
• Can you see the tube bisect the carina?
• Can you see the tube cross the diaphragm in the midline?
• Does the tube then deviate immediately to the left?
• Can you see the tip of the tube clearly below the left hemidiaphragm?
• If you think the tube is in the esophagus, can you advance it?
• Has the tube coiled higher up in the pharynx or esophagus?
• Does the length of tube inserted suggest it should be in the stomach?
• Does the X-ray image cover enough of the area below the diaphragm to enable you to see the tube clearly, or does it need to be repeated?

Source: Adapted from reference 22.

tube should be inside the stomach, but misplacement is common (Table 5.2 and Figure 5.2).[22] Discomfort at the oropharyngeal insertion site can be improved with an anesthetic gel.[3] The tolerance of nasogastric feeding is determined by gastric residual volumes. Careful evaluation of abdominal bowel sounds and abdominal girth or serial abdominal radiographs to look for air or fluid levels are necessary to determine adequate gastrointestinal function.

Gastric residual volumes in the range of 200 to 500 mL are problematic and indicative of gastric dysfunction. In these patients, abdominal distension may occur, and enteral nutrition may have to be discontinued; but there is uncertainty on how much gastric residual volume can be tolerated before enteral feeding is stopped (Table 5.3).

Gastric motility is commonly abnormal in bedbound patients and may simply be a response to sympathetic stimulation associated with any type of injury, in particular neurologic injury. The effect of this motility abnormality can be protracted and may last several days. In addition, drugs such as opioids, β-adrenergic agents, and α-2 agonists all significantly impact on gastric emptying, as do metabolic derangements such as hyperglycemia, hypoglycemia, hypermagnesemia, metabolic acidosis, and sepsis.

Most patients who are acutely ill may enter an area of partial starvation that leads to loss of lean body mass, which may predispose them to further infections and other complications. The caloric intake rapidly declines, and deficit usually occurs in the first week of admission. There is no proven benefit of early parenteral nutrition to improve caloric intake or to achieve caloric intake or to reduce length of stay in the intensive care unit or duration of artificial ventilation.

Table 5.3 **Solutions for gastric retention and diarrhea**

Gastric Residual Volume >500 mL
• Initiate metoclopramide 10 mg IV q 6 hours
• Initiate naloxone 8 mg in saline per tube q 6 hours
• Turn patient to right lateral decubitus position
Gastric Residual Volume >500 mL
• Hold enteral infusion
• Restart infusion once GRV <500 mL
• Recheck GRV in 2 hours
Diarrhea (>250 mL/day stool output per rectum or >1,000 mL/day output per ileostomy)
• Remove sorbitol from oral/enteric medications
• Obtain stool cultures/toxin assays to rule out infectious diarrhea
• Consider fiber-containing formula or small peptide/MCT formula
• Consider opiates once infectious etiology ruled out

GRV = gastric residual volume; MCT = medium-chain triglyceride. (From reference 20.)

Parenteral nutritional solutions are easily available and designed to meet patient needs. If enteral feeding is not feasible. Total parenteral nutrition (TPN) feeding according to guidelines includes 7% amino acid, 10%–20% glucose, and 22 kcal/kg IBW. This will avoid overfeeding. Large quantities of dextrose—easily administered through TPN—may cause significant hyperglycemia and should be avoided. Protein requirements are typically about 1.5 g/kg per day, but in patients with insufficient caloric intake, protein in doses of 2.0 to 3.5 g/kg per day is recommended. Fat must be provided in 500-mL aliquots of 10% emulsion, and the total dose of calories must be less than 60% of the total nonprotein calories. The basic components are: (1) dextrose 50%, which provides 250 g in a 500-mL solution; (2) amino acid mixture of 8.5% in 500-mL bottles; and (3) 10% fat emulsion in 500-mL bottles. The formula is supplemented with standard electrolyte solutions, daily multivitamins, and trace elements.

As mentioned earlier, gastric residuals should be <200 mL: only then does it appear that there is satisfactory feeding. If the gastric residual is >500 mL, erythromycin 250 mg q.i.d. is started. This may be supplemented with metoclopramide 10–20 mg q.i.d., and both drugs should reduce residuals. If this remains unsuccessful, a nasojejunal tube should be placed. Persistent residuals should be investigated carefully with an abdominal X-ray for paralytic ileus. Absolute contraindications to enteral nutrition are evidence of gut obstruction, gut failure due to extensive resection or absorption impairment, and acute pancreatitis.

Typically nutrition reaches its goal of 80% requirement within 72 hours.

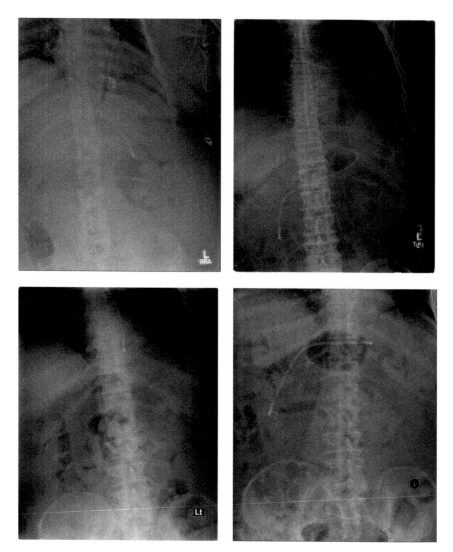

Figure 5.2 Common positions of nasogastric tube (upper row (correct): mid gastric, postpyloric; lower row (incorrect): esophageal, and descending duodenum.

The standard enteral nutrition formulas also deliver approximately 50% of calories as carbohydrates and 0.33% as fat. Protein is delivered in a content of approximately 40 g/L. Fiber is often added to improve diarrhea or constipation.[15,16] Continuous gastric feeds are typically best tolerated. Intensive care unit trials show no differences between continuous versus bolus feeding.[23]

Problems with feeding are generally diarrhea, inability to meet nutritional targets, inability to maintain nasogastric tube in situ, and obstructing tubes.[29,40]

Diarrhea is common and can be changed by increasing fiber and changing to a different enteral nutrition. Electrolytes should be aggressively replaced. *Clostridium difficile* or *Enterobacter* needs to be excluded in most patients but is rarely a cause of diarrhea. Often the delivery of nutrition through the nasogastric route is then changed to transpyloric feeding tubes but several studies have not been able to find better nutrition as a result of postpyloric feeding.

A common problem is continuation of medication by this route, but absorption should be sufficient for most drugs. Specific absorption problems have been noted with warfarin, phenytoin, and carbamazepine. Absorption of phenytoin with tube feeding is poor, in some patients virtually immeasurable. One method is to hold feeding 2 hours before administration. This should result in adequate absorption and therapeutic phenytoin plasma levels, but the total dose may still need to be increased.

The decision to proceed with percutaneous endoscopic gastrostomy (PEG) is related to how long nasogastric feeding may need to continue. Most nutritionists feel that the PEG placement should be considered if there is more than 4 weeks of anticipated abnormal swallowing mechanism or gastric motility disorder, but this cannot be accurately assessed clinically in most instances. PEG placement has been studied in many neurologic disorders including stroke, traumatic brain injury, and the more common acute and chronic neuromuscular diseases. Risk of complications with PEG placement is very low at less than 0.5%. It may cause a localized infection and gastric hemorrhage. Air under diaphragm on Chest X ray is common after placement and should not be interpreted as a potential complication.

PEG is considered in any acute neuromuscular disorder that requires long-term mechanical ventilation and is combined with a tracheostomy. PEG placement in ALS patients may be associated with complications due to their previous poor nutritional status, and we have had patients with hypotension and transient worsening respiratory function with this procedure.[33]

Refeeding syndrome is another concern that has been described in many conditions; in ALS it is due to long-term dysphagia resulting from poor nutrition. Patients with prolonged vomiting and malnourished alcoholics are also at major risk of refeeding syndrome; in fact, any patient with no substantial feeding for 7 days is at risk. This syndrome causes major electrolyte abnormalities such as hypophosphatemia, hypokalemia, hypomagnesemia, hyperglycemia, and thiamine deficiency, all due to increased demand with feeding. Clinically this may lead to muscular weakness and respiratory failure or prolonged weaning, cardiac arrhythmias, or at its extreme the development of Wernicke encephalopathy. These deficiencies can be replaced with NaPhos, KPhos, magnesium sulfate, and intravenous KCl. Several measurements of serum phosphate are needed to prove stable laboratory findings.[13,31,41,42]

By the Way

Feeding Formulas

- Osmolite is an isotonic standard house formula
- Osmolite 1.5 and TwoCal HN are calorie dense
- Promote is high-protein formula
- Jevity has high fiber content per liter

Nutrition by the Numbers

- ~60% of patients with chronic diabetes have gastric emptying problems
- ~40% of patients are malnourished
- ~30% of hospitalized patients may have serious weight loss
- ~25% less calories increases risk for poor outcome
- ~20% of US adults have a metabolic syndrome
- ~10% of ICU patients could develop refeeding syndrome with nutrition

---

Putting It All Together

- Early feeding reduces complications and even mortality
- Underfeeding is just as worrisome as overfeeding
- Sick patients require 25% additional calories but not >30 kcal/kg IBW
- Enteral feeding should not lead to >500 mL retention
- Diarrhea is common and may improve with changing nutrition formula
- PEG is often considered early and are usually 10 days after admission in mechanically ventilated patients

References

1. Alberda C, Gramlich L, Jones N, et al. The relationship between nutritional intake and clinical outcomes in critically ill patients: results of an international multicenter observational study. *Intensive Care Med* 2009;35:1728–1737.
2. Artinian V, Krayem H, DiGiovine B. Effects of early enteral feeding on the outcome of critically ill mechanically ventilated medical patients. *Chest* 2006;129:960–967.
3. Banerjee TS, Schneider HJ. Recommended method of attachment of nasogastric tubes. *Ann R Coll Surg Engl* 2007;89:529–530.
4. Berger MM. Analyzing ICU physician and dietitian adherence to nutrition therapy guidelines. *JPEN J Parenter Enteral Nutr* 2010;34:606–607.
5. Blackburn GL, Wollner S, Bistrian BR. Nutrition support in the intensive care unit: an evolving science. *Arch Surg* 2010;145:533–538.

6. Collier BR, Giladi A, Dossett LA, Dyer L, Fleming SB, Cotton BA. Impact of high-dose antioxidants on outcomes in acutely injured patients. *JPEN J Parenter Enteral Nutr* 2008;32:384–388.
7. Davidson JE, Kruse MW, Cox DH, Duncan R. Critical care of the morbidly obese. *Crit Care Nurs Q* 2003;26:105–116.
8. Debaveye Y, Van den Berghe G. Risks and benefits of nutritional support during critical illness. *Annu Rev Nutr* 2006;26:513–538.
9. Doig GS, Heighes PT, Simpson F, Sweetman EA, Davies AR. Early enteral nutrition, provided within 24 h of injury or intensive care unit admission, significantly reduces mortality in critically ill patients: a meta-analysis of randomized controlled trials. *Intensive Care Med* 2009;35:2018–2027.
10. Doig GS, Heighes PT, Simpson F, Sweetman EA. Early enteral nutrition reduces mortality in trauma patients requiring intensive care: a meta-analysis of randomised controlled trials. *Injury* 2011;42:50–56.
11. Doig GS, Simpson F, Finfer S, et al. Effect of evidence-based feeding guidelines on mortality of critically ill adults: a cluster randomized controlled trial. *JAMA* 2008;300:2731–2741.
12. Fabbri A, Magrini N, Bianchi G, Zoli M, Marchesini G. Overview of randomized clinical trials of oral branched-chain amino acid treatment in chronic hepatic encephalopathy. *J Parenter Enteral Nutr* 1996;20:159–164.
13. Gentile MG, Pastorelli P, Ciceri R, et al. Specialized refeeding treatment for anorexia nervosa patients suffering from extreme undernutrition. *Clin Nutr* 2010;29:627–632.
14. Gottschlich MM. *The A.S.P.E.N Nutrition Support Core Curriculum: A Case-Based Approach; The Adult Patient.* Silver Spring (MD), American Society for Parenteral and Enteral Nutrition, 2007.
15. Gupta B, Agrawal P, Soni KD, et al. Enteral nutrition practices in the intensive care unit: understanding of nursing practices and perspectives. *J Anaesthesiol Clin Pharmacol* 2012;28:41–44.
16. Hayes GL, McKinzie BP, Bullington WM, Cooper TB, Pilch NA. Nutritional supplements in critical illness. *AACN Adv Crit Care* 2011;22:301–316.
17. Heyland DK, Dhaliwal R, Drover JW, et al. Canadian clinical practice guidelines for nutrition support in mechanically ventilated, critically ill adult patients. *JPEN J Parenter Enteral Nutr* 2003;27:355–373.
18. Heyland DK, Dhaliwal R, Drover JW, Gramlich L, Dodek P; Canadian Critical Care Clinical Practice Guidelines Committee. Canadian clinical practice guidelines for nutrition support in mechanically ventilated, critically ill adult patients. *JPEN J Parenter Enteral Nutr* 2003;27:355–373.
19. Honiden S, McArdle JR. Obesity in the intensive care unit. *Clin Chest Med* 2009;30:581–599.
20. Kondrup J, Allison SP, Elia M, et al. ESPEN guidelines for nutrition screening 2002. *Clin Nutr* 2003;22:415–421.
21. Kreymann KG, Berger MM, Deutz NE, et al. ESPEN guidelines on enteral nutrition: intensive care. *Clin Nutr* 2006;25:210–223.
22. Lamont T, Beaumont C, Fayaz A, et al. Checking placement of nasogastric feeding tubes in adults (interpretation of x ray images): summary of a safety report from the National Patient Safety Agency. *BMJ* 2011;342:d2586.
23. MacLeod JB, Lefton J, Houghton D, et al. Prospective randomized control trial of intermittent versus continuous gastric feeds for critically ill trauma patients. *J Trauma* 2007;63:57–61.
24. Manzanares W, Hardy G. Thiamine supplementation in the critically ill. *Curr Opin Clin Nutr Metab Care* 2012;14:610–617.
25. Marik PE, Zaloga GP. Early enteral nutrition in acutely ill patients: a systematic review. *Crit Care Med* 2001;29:2264–2270.
26. Martindale RG, McCarthy MS, McClave SA. Guidelines for nutrition therapy in critical illness: are not they all the same? *Minerva Anestesiol* 2011;77:463–467.
27. Martindale RG, McClave SA, Vanek VW, et al. Guidelines for the provision and assessment of nutrition support therapy in the adult critically ill patient: Society of Critical Care

Medicine and American Society for Parenteral and Enteral Nutrition: Executive Summary. *Crit Care Med* 2009;37:1757–1761.

28. McClave SA, Martindale RG, Vanek VW, et al. Guidelines for the provision and assessment of nutrition support therapy in the adult critically ill patient: Society of Critical Care Medicine (SCCM) and American Society for Parenteral and Enteral Nutrition (A.S.P.E.N.). *JPEN J Parenter Enteral Nutr* 2009;33:277–316.

29. McGinnis CM, Worthington P, Lord LM. Nasogastric versus feeding tubes in critically ill patients. *Crit Care Nurse* 2010;30:80–82.

30. Mechanick JI, Chiolero R. Special commentary: a call for intensive metabolic support. *Curr Opin Clin Nutr Metab Care* 2008;11:666–670.

31. Mehanna HM, Moledina J, Travis J. Refeeding syndrome: what is it, and how to prevent and treat it. *BJM* 2008;336:1495–1498.

32. Miller KR, Kiraly LN, Lowen CC, Martindale RG, McClave SA. "CAN WE FEED?" A mnemonic to merge nutrition and intensive care assessment of the critically ill patient. *JPEN J Parenter Enteral Nutr* 2011;35:643–659.

33. Miller RG, Jackson CE, Kasarskis EJ, et al.; Quality Standards Subcommittee of the American Academy of Neurology. Practice parameter update: the care of the patient with amyotrophic lateral sclerosis: multidisciplinary care, symptom management, and cognitive/behavioral impairment (an evidence-based review): report of the Quality Standards Subcommittee of the American Academy of Neurology. *Neurology* 2009;73:1227–1233.

34. Passier RH, Davies AR, Ridley E, McClure J, Murphy D, Scheinkestel CD. Periprocedural cessation of nutrition in the intensive care unit: opportunities for improvement. *Intensive Care Med* 2013;39:1221–1226.

35. Port AM, Apovian C. Metabolic support of the obese intensive care unit patient: a current perspective. *Curr Opin Clin Nutr Metab Care* 2010;13:184–191.

36. Simpson F, Doig GS. Parenteral vs. enteral nutrition in the critically ill patient: a meta-analysis of trials using the intention to treat principle. *Intensive Care Med* 2005;31:12–23.

37. Singer P, Anbar R, Cohen J, et al. The tight calorie control study (TICACOS): a prospective, randomized, controlled pilot study of nutritional support in critically ill patients. *Intensive Care Med* 2011;37:601–609.

38. Stroud M. Protein and the critically ill: do we know what to give? *Proc Nutr Soc* 2007;66:378–383.

39. Thomas DR. Causes of protein-calorie malnutrition. *Z Gerontol Geriatr* 1999;32 Supp 1:I38–144.

40. Thibault R, Graf S, Clerc A, Delieuvin N, Heidegger CP, Pichard C. Diarrhea in the ICU: respective contribution of feeding and antibiotics. *Crit Care* 2013;24;17:R153.

41. Tresley J, Sheean PM. Refeeding syndrome: recognition is the key to prevention and management. *J Am Diet Assoc* 2008;108:2105–2108.

42. Weisinger JR, Bellorin-Font E. Magnesium and phosphorus. *Lancet* 1998;352:391–396.

6

Fluid and Electrolyte Monitoring

Maintenance of an effective circulating volume, supplementing electrolytes, and correcting an acid-base imbalance are important goals in any hospitalized patient, but more so in an acutely ill neurologic patient and there distinguishing features. Acutely ill neurologic patients admitted to hospital wards or intensive care units can be expected to have a marginal fluid balance or may be dehydrated. Once in the hospital, daily data on fluid intake and output are often helpful, albeit inaccurate and not always adjusted to the patient's needs. Adequate fluid resuscitation—in the broadest sense—is reflected by normal blood pressure and normal urinary output. Thus, hypovolemia (and hypotension) leads to tachycardia, oliguria and, eventually, increased blood urea nitrogen (BUN), increased serum lactate and acidosis from poor tissue perfusion. Acute brain injury could impair thirst mechanisms, and as a result the patient may not gain access to fluids. If adequate fluids are not provided, water loss may lead to an increase of serum sodium and osmolality. Some patients may already be off to a bad start if osmotic agents to treat brain swelling have been administered. Furthermore, any acute physiologic stress response results in dysregulating the normal homeostatic mechanism, which leads to conservation of water and salt because acute brain injury stimulates the sympathetic nervous system and the renin-angiotensin system. This competing mechanism may cause problems if additional fluids are administered and, therefore, can easily tip the balance to fluid overload.

There are more differences that set acute ill neurologic patients apart from the rest. Electrolyte abnormalities are ubiquitous and mostly related to illness-associated electrolyte loss or inability to maintain adequate water balance.[44] Acute changes in sodium homeostasis may also cause changes in brain water. The type of replacement fluid therapy is particularly important in acutely ill neurologic patients and particularly hypotonic fluids could worsen brain edema.

It is necessary to monitor and manage fluids and electrolytes daily. The most urgent questions are: Is the patient well hydrated? Are electrolytes replaced? Are the electrolyte abnormalities a consequence of an abnormal fluid balance and fluid intake? Are there changes in acid-base balance that need correction? This chapter provides the essentials of management and how to interpret concerning values.

Principles

The regimen for normal maintenance of fluid intake is based on an estimation of fluid losses and must be carefully monitored by laboratory measurements. These laboratory investigations should include daily serum electrolytes, osmolality, creatinine, BUN, serum glucose, and, when indicated, an arterial blood gas. Theoretically weighing the patient could provide some sense of net gain or loss of fluid, but because fluid balance on the wards—and even in more monitored setting and intensive care units—is far from reliable. Body weight variations also have more to do with measurement errors than with changes in fluid balance.

A first principle concerns the administration of intravenous fluids through a peripheral access using a large-bore (18-gauge) needle to allow blood products and large volumes of fluids. Starting with isotonic saline (0.9% sodium chloride) would provide sufficient sodium intake. In most patients an initial fluid intake of 150–200 mL/h is appropriate, but remember that kidneys are better at conserving water than washing out. Dextrose-based solutions should have no place in patients with acute neurologic disorders unless a severe hypernatremia needs correction. Dextrose stimulates release of insulin and also promotes potassium entering into cells, which can lead to hyperkalemia. Large volumes of dextrose-containing solutions may also further worsen hyperglycemia. Hyperglycemia and anaerobic cerebral glucose metabolism result in toxic accumulation of lactate and intracellular acidosis, which in turn may set off lipid peroxidation and free radical formation (Chapter 7).

A second principle is that serum sodium is an important marker of fluid balance. Hyponatremia is mostly a relative water surplus in relation to the quantity of intravascular sodium. Conversely, hypernatremia is mostly a relative water deficit in relation to the quantity of intravascular sodium. Thus to treat hyponatremia, one should use a more concentrated fluid concentration, switching from 0.9% sodium chloride to 1.5% sodium chloride. In the treatment of hypernatremia, the solution should become more dilute and switched to 0.45% sodium chloride, lactated Ringer's or, in extreme hypernatremia, 5% dextrose.

A third principle is that body water, is best understood as different fluid compartments.[21] The extracellular fluid compartment consists of intervascular and interstitial spaces. The intervascular compartment is about 10% of total body weight. Physiologic principles maintain that water distribution in the body is largely determined by osmotic forces; therefore, change in osmolality can change water movement across cell membranes. These osmotic differences are determined by sodium and potassium, which cannot cross the cell membrane and are therefore effective osmoles.

The glomerular afferent arteriole and specialized renal cells that regulate activity of the renin-angiotensin system, and the changes in fluid homeostasis and its corrective measures, are shown in Figure 6.1. A rise in plasma osmolality leads to an increase in antidiuretic hormone (ADH) secretion. This will limit urinary water losses and return the osmolality to normal. This also requires increased water intake through thirst or administration through fluids. A decrease in plasma

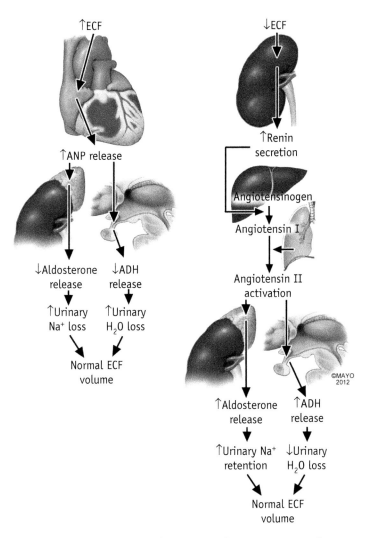

Figure 6.1 Endocrine responses to changes in volume status in order to maintain homeostasis.

osmolality, for example, after abundant free water administration, reduces ADH release and permits excretion of excess water. Apparently the system responds to less than 2% variability in plasma osmolality and is usually determined by the concentration of the major plasma solutes. The equation is:

$$\text{Plasma osmolality} = 2 \times \text{serum sodium} + \frac{\text{serum glucose}}{18} + \frac{\text{BUN}}{2.8}$$
$$= 275 - 295\,\text{mOsm} / \text{kg}$$

A fourth principle is to understand the fundamentals of fluid administration. Fluid resuscitation includes crystalloids (electrolyte-based solution) or colloids (large-molecular-weight solutions). It is not known whether isotonic or hypertonic fluids are different in their efficacy in fluid resuscitation or which one produces a better result.[36] Crystalloids are solutions in which sodium is the major osmotically active particle (e.g., isotonic saline, lactated Ringer's solution, hypertonic saline). The most commonly used crystalloid is 0.9% sodium chloride or normal saline. This solution is slightly hypertonic to plasma (308 mOsm/kg as opposed to plasma osmolality of 289 mOsm/kg). The distribution of this fluid when administered will follow the normal rule of proportions and, thus, only 100–250 mL for every liter will remain in the intravascular compartment. (Remember that plasma volume makes up only 3 liters of the 14 liters of extracellular volume.)

Colloids work through a mechanism of changing the intravascular plasma colloid osmotic pressure that normally is in balance with interstitial colloid osmotic pressure. Colloid solutions change the blood rheology, reduce viscosity, and improve blood flow. Albumin can be an effective resuscitation solution.[20] The large molecules cannot pass the capillary membrane and then start acting as a potential sponge. The volume administered intravascularly does not distribute. Thus, 250 mL isosmotic colloids (5% albumin) results in an approximately 250 mL change in intravascular volume. Only hyperosmotic solutions (25% albumin) will draw far more into the intravascular system. Albumin 5% eventually expands intravascular volume by only 15 mL of water per gram, but albumin 25% expands intravascular volume five times more than the infused volume. Again this difference is explained by a much higher colloid osmotic pressure, the major determinant of fluid distribution. The effect of both types of albumin lasts at least 24 hours. Still, most of total body albumin moves into the extravascular compartment. This is also expected with hypertonic crystalloids (3% NaCl, 7.5% NaCl, 23% NaCl). When 250 mL of 7.5% sodium chloride is administered, the intravascular volume will increase three- to four-fold due to its water-indrawing osmotic effect.

The major advantages of fluid replacement with colloids are a smaller infused volume, prolonged plasma expansion, and minimal peripheral edema. The major disadvantage is that hemostasis may be not be as effective as a result of reduced factor VIII activity and increased fibrinolysis. Anaphylaxis with cardiorespiratory arrest has been reported with albumin but is very uncommon.[28,40]

How about the age-old Ringer's solution? Isotonic lactated Ringer's contains lactate, more potassium, and less sodium, therefore causing potential hypervolemia and worsening hyponatremia in patients with acute brain injury already predisposed to hyponatremia. It also causes metabolic alkalosis with large volumes. Lactated Ringer's solution, an electrolyte solution used frequently in patients with polytrauma, is slightly hypotonic (273 mOsm/kg). Hypotonic solutions—again tonicity reflects sodium concentration—such as "half-normal" saline (0.45 NaCl) or 5% dextrose in water (D5W) provides nearly free (free meaning free of electrolytes) water.

In Practice

Fluid administration is always fluctuating and never constant. Increased fluid requirements are needed in patients with nasogastric suction, diuretics, vomiting, diarrhea, glycosuria, diabetes insipidus, hyperventilation, excessive sweating, hyperthyroidism, and, most commonly, fever. Decreased requirements are needed in patients with heart and kidney failure, hypoalbuminemia, and evidence of fluid overload. Urinary output is a good guide, and 40 cc/h is adequate.

Usually an initial fluid intake of 150–200 mL/h is appropriate. Administration can go through a peripheral venous catheter. Hypertonic solutions (starting already with 3% saline and up) need a central access to prevent severe phlebitis, which may occur already with a single administered bolus. Access can be provided through a peripherally inserted central catheter (PICC) or an internal jugular (IJ) catheter.

FLUID RESUSCITATION IN PRACTICE

How do we define hypovolemia? Hypovolemia may occur from hemorrhage, rapid loss from vomiting, or excessive sweating. Loss of fluids may be due to "third spacing," defined as fluid located in the interstitial space or peritoneal cavity in edema or ascites. Third spacing strictly means disproportionately more fluids in these locations than in the intracellular or extracellular volume. Decreased intravascular volume results in corrective measures; but before that, blood pressure may decline to systolic blood pressure less than 90 mm Hg. Tachycardia from a sympathetic response and peripheral vasoconstriction and retention of sodium and water result in oliguria. Laboratory tests are showing hypernatremia, increased creatinine and blood urea nitrogen, decreased hemoglobin (from possible fluid resuscitation or due to hemorrhage), hyperglycemia, increased lactate, and decreased pH from tissue acidosis.

Adding the hourly urine output to the patient's insensible loss, which is estimated at 30–50 mL/h, is a way to simply calculate the rate of fluid administration. If necessary, 1–2 liters of isotonic saline can be immediately administered in patients who are volume depleted or are in a true hypovolemic shock. A positive fluid balance can be achieved if the administration of fluid is at a rate that is 50–100 mL/h greater than estimated fluid losses.

What are the current views on how best to resuscitate the patient when needed? Resuscitation protocols have shifted dramatically over the last years, and known techniques such as active rewarming and aggressive blood product administration have changed.[13,15,38] Permissive hypotension has emerged in trauma resuscitation. The overriding concern is that with significant restoration of blood pressure, bleeding may be facilitated and may worsen the patient through uncontrolled hemorrhagic shock. Many trauma resuscitation protocols include acceptance of a mean arterial pressure (MAP) of 50–65 mmHg. Such MAP values may be too low for patients with acute brain injury. Another new approach is so-called balance transfusion, providing red blood cells and fresh frozen plasma in a ratio of 1 unit of red blood cells to 1 unit of fresh frozen plasma.

Crystalloids are the best fluid therapy. In a hypotensive patient, fluid resuscitation restores blood pressure when there is a volume deficit. However, the clinical condition may be associated with a vasodilatory state (i.e., sepsis); and large amounts of fluids may be rapidly administered without much effect on blood pressure other than a rapid fluid overload. Fluid overload may lead to pulmonary edema (impaired gas exchange), gut edema (ileus), and increased renal venous pressure (reduced glomerulofiltration rate and uremia). Early use of vasopressor (norepinephrine or vasopressin infusion) is far more beneficial than previously thought. If liberal fluid resuscitation is defined as fluid replacement of 3–5 liters, then conservative replacement of 1–3 liters may still be very effective in restoring adequate intravascular volume.

SODIUM ABNORMALITIES

Hyponatremia is quite common in hospitalized patients and thus also in neurologic patients.[12,27,32,45,48] It occurs in nearly half of patients with aneurysmal subarachnoid hemorrhage, a large proportion of patients with bacterial meningitis, and also in patients with severe traumatic brain injury.

Serum sodium usually declines several days following the acute brain injury and is seldom severe.[8] Values between 120–130 mmol/L are typical. Because hyponatremia is most often a reflection of a change in volume status, it has been traditionally stratified according to volume status[43] (Figure 6.2). Hyponatremia and hypovolemia can occur as a result of gastrointestinal and renal losses. Hyponatremia and normovolemia can occur with no dietary salt

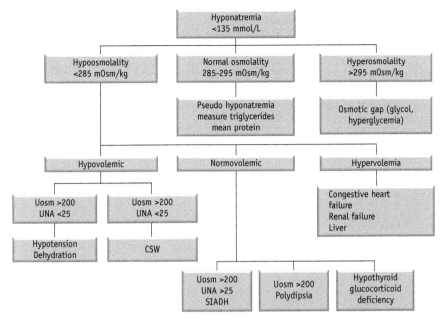

Figure 6.2 Evaluation of hyponatremia by volume status. CSW: Cerebral salt wasting, SIADH: Inappropriate antidiuretic hormone secretion.

intake, low glucocorticoid status, or hypothyroidism.[11,25,37] Hypervolemia is typically seen in congestive heart failure or liver cirrhosis, but also in patients with advanced renal failure. Acute dilutional hyponatremia to values less than 110 mEq/L is most concerning. In acute dilutional hyponatremia associated with hypoosmolality, brain swelling could occur from water gain due to the osmotic gradient. It is corrected within hours by cellular loss of sodium, potassium, chloride, and water (a rapid adaptation). The hypoosmolar state is corrected gradually (within days) through loss of so-called osmolytes. These extruded "idiogenic osmols" are solutes such as glutamate, glutamine, taurine, and myoinositol, but the transcription of genes coding for activation of transporters takes time (a slow adaptation). The brain adaptation to hyperosmolality is not the reverse, and in acute hyperosmolality, rapid electrolyte accumulation from cerebrospinal fluid, plasma, and extracellular fluid results in correction of intracellular brain water.

Cerebral salt wasting is a deficiency of salt. In syndrome of inappropriate antidiuretic hormone secretion (SIADH) the volume expansion suppresses aldosterone and increases natriuretic peptides leading to hypertonic high sodium containing urine and retention of relatively electrolyte free water eventually resulting in hyponatremia.[45] The presence of high urinary sodium content in both conditions does not distinguish between cerebral salt wasting syndrome and SIADH, and there is no other laboratory difference between the two. The only difference is volume status. There is volume depletion in cerebral salt wasting syndrome and a

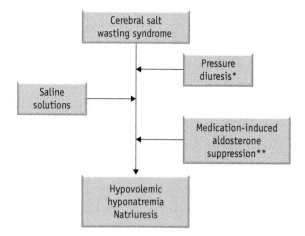

Figure 6.3 Major confounders in cerebral salt wasting syndrome.
*Increased symphathetic activity; inotropes, vasopressors. **calcium-channel blockers, inotropes such as dopamine.

normal or expanded volume status in SIADH. SIADH should be treated with fluid restriction and a loop diuretic. Hypovolemic hyponatremia responds to hypertonic saline causing more dilute urine after vasopressin drops (due to correction of hypovolemia) and serum sodium rises after loss of water. Cerebral salt wasting is often confounded by other interventions and may not be seen in its purest form (Figure 6.3).

In hospitalized patients, the most important factor associated with hospital-acquired hyponatremia remains the administration of hypotonic fluids. Thiazide diuretics are well known to cause hyponatremia due to impaired urinary diluting capacity.

The treatment of hyponatremia typically consists of increased sodium content in intravenous fluid, addition of a mineralocorticoid, increased salt intake with the use of high-salt-containing liquids such as V8, and free water restriction.[8,23,33] The optimal rate of correction of severe hyponatremia is the correction of no more than 6 mEq/L/day and within 6 hours to correct the most severe hyponatremia.[45] The formula proposed by Adrogue and Madias estimates the effect of any infusate on serum, and calculators are available (www.medcalc. com).[6] Generally an infusion of 1 mL/kg of 3% saline (540 mEq NaCL) will raise serum sodium by approximately 1 mEq/L. In these patients, serum sodium needs to be checked every 2 hours. It has also been suggested to treat acute severe hyponatremia (causing seizures and coma) with a 100 mL bolus of 3% saline with two extra doses every 15 minutes if neurologic condition does not improve.[45]

In patients with hypernatremia, the first task is to determine whether hypernatremia is the result of dehydration or excessive sodium, but hypernatremia can occur in states of euvolemia or hypervolemia. One cause of increased total body sodium is excess administration of hypertonic sodium bicarbonate to correct metabolic acidosis.[3,5,7,30,31] In addition, with the increased and repeated use of hypertonic sodium solutions to treat increased intracranial pressure, hypernatremia is expected.[17] Failure to replace insensible losses and failure to adjust intravenous fluids remain the most common causes of hypernatremia in sick patients. Also, in severe acute brain injury, central diabetes insipidus may be a factor and further tests are needed.[19] The diagnosis is supported if the urine is hypotonic (urine osmolality < 300 mOsm/kg, urine specific gravity < 1.010) despite hypertonic serum (plasma osmolality >300 mOsm/kg).

The majority of patients with hypernatremia are hypovolemic, requiring isotonic or hypotonic saline. Fluid resuscitation in patients with hypernatremia usually involves switching to a 0.45% NaCl infusion using a rate correction formula (www.medcalc.com).[5] Diabetes insipidus, with serum sodium greater than 160 mmol/L, can be treated with desmopressin 1 mcg IV, followed by additional doses as needed to normalize the serum sodium. Free water flushes through the nasogastric tube can be used if hypernatremia is stable and less than 150 mmol/L.

POTASSIUM ABNORMALITIES

Most critically ill patients have hypokalemia at some stage in their clinical course, and often there is more than one reason for potassium deficiency. Common causes for hypokalemia are gastrointestinal problems, skin losses, or drugs. The development of metabolic alkalosis from nasogastric suctioning may also cause an increase in renal potassium excretion. When the serum potassium level decreases (<3 mEq/L), total body potassium stores most likely are significantly depleted, and electrocardiographic changes are often seen. Prominent U waves, ST-segment changes, dampened T wave, and, more important, atrial and ventricular arrhythmias could point to a more rapidly developing severe hypokalemia.[22]

Patients with severe hypokalemia have a mild degree of rhabdomyolysis. The mechanism of rhabdomyolysis in severe hypokalemia is not known. In this context, rhabdomyolysis is not significant enough to result in its classic presentations of compartment syndrome or acute tubular necrosis. Widespread muscle pain that may have started in the calves is present. Muscles are firmly swollen and extremely tender to touch. Many patients complain of intensifying pain with movement.

Hyperkalemia is most commonly encountered in patients with renal or adrenal failure.[9,47] Hyperkalemia has also been anecdotally described in patients on cardiac bypass. In these patients, increased plasma potassium may be induced by washout of ischemic underperfused areas during the body's bypass period or may be caused by rewarming after hypothermia. Treatment of hypokalemia and hyperkalemia is shown in Tables 6.1 and 6.2.

Table 6.1 **Treatment of Hypokalemia**

Severity	Serum Potassium Concentration (mEq/L)	IV Potassium Replacement Dose (mEq)
Mild to moderate	2.5–3.4	20–40
Severe	<2.5	40–80

Source: From reference 22.

Table 6.2 **Treatments for Hyperkalemia**

Treatment	Dose	Route	Time to Onset	Duration of Effect
Calcium gluconate	1–2 g (4.56–9.12 mEq calcium)	IV over 5–10 min	1–2 min	10–30 min
Sodium bicarbonate	50–100 mEq	IV over 2–5 min	30 min	2–6 h
Insulin (regular) (with dextrose)	5–10 units	IV with 50 mL of 50% dextrose injection	15–45 min	2–6 h
50% dextrose	50 mL (25 g)	IV over 5 min	30 min	2–6 h
10% dextrose	1,000 mL (100 g)	IV over 5 min	30 min	2–6 h

Source: From reference 22.

MAGNESIUM, PHOSPHATE, AND CALCIUM ABNORMALITIES

Other electrolytes that are commonly abnormal are hypomagnesemia and hypophosphatemia.[42] Hypomagnesemia is often detected in hospitalized patients. It can be related to ventricular arrhythmias and therefore is important to correct.[4,39] Normally magnesium depletion results in marked reduction of magnesium excretion by the kidneys; however, renal magnesium wasting can occur with diuretics, aminoglycosides, or certain chemotherapeutic agents. It is not uncommonly seen in patients with long-standing diarrhea associated with nasogastric feeding, hypocalcemia, or refractory hypokalemia. Potassium-sparing diuretics might be necessary in patients who have hypomagnesemia associated with a thiazide or loop diuretic. Most of the time, magnesium is easily corrected by maintaining the plasma magnesium concentration above 1.0 mg/dL using 50 μEq of IV magnesium given slowly over 8 hours (Table 6.3).[14,39]

Hypophosphatemia is common during illness, when phosphate stores are easily depleted.[20,24,41] Most likely causes of hypophosphatemia in hospital patients are prior chronic diarrhea or chronic antacid intake. It is also more common if the patient has received insulin infusion to correct hyperglycemia. Treatment is typically in asymptomatic patients with a serum phosphate level <2.0 mg/dL, and oral dosing might be sufficient. Oral phosphate supplements include 250 mg

Table 6.3 **Treatment of Hypomagnesemia**

Severity	Serum Magnesium Concentration (mg/dL)	IV Magnesium Replacement Dose
Mild to moderate	1.0–1.5	8–32 mEq magnesium (1–4 g magnesium sulfate), up to 1.0 mEq/kg
Severe	<1.0	32–64 mEq magnesium (4–8 g magnesium sulfate), up to 1.5 mEq/kg

Source: From reference 2.

Table 6.4 **Treatment of Hypophosphatemia**

Serum Phosphorus Concentration (mg/dL)	IV Phosphate Replacement Dose (mmol/kg)
2.3–2.7	0.08–0.16
1.5–2.2	0.16–0.32
<1.5	0.32–0.64

Source: From reference 41.

of phosphate. Intravenous administration of phosphate is another way to cor-rect hypophosphatemia and is shown in Table 6.4. An aggressive approach is only needed in patients who receive nutritional support, and in this setting infusion is recommended at 7.5 mmol/hour.[29] Switching to oral replacement is recommended when the serum phosphate concentration reaches 1.5 mg/dL. Hyperphosphatemia is mostly seen in renal failure but may occur with parenteral nutrition. Treatment is using phosphate binders shown in Table 6.5.

Calcium abnormalities can be seen in acutely ill neurologic patients but mostly in more critically ill conditions such as sepsis, pancreatitis but also in multitrauma patients with crush injury. Hypocalcemia may cause seizures of less than 3 mEq/L. Most of the time hypocalcemia is a result of chronic illness and easily supplemented (Table 6.6).[10]

ACID-BASE DISORDERS

The basic pathophysiology of acid-base disorders is very predictable, but complex or mixed disorders often occur. Acid-base disorder analysis can be simplified and requires pH, $PaCO_2$, and HCO_3. Respiratory acidosis and alkalosis result primar-ily in changes in arterial PCO_2; metabolic acidosis and alkalosis result primarily in changes in HCO_3. Metabolic acidosis or metabolic alkalosis results in pH and $PaCO_2$ in the same direction. Respiratory alkalosis and respiratory acidosis result in pH or $PaCO_2$ in opposite directions. The pH and $PaCO_2$ change in opposite

Table 6.5 **Treatment of Hyperphosphatemia**

Medication	Dosage Forms	Initial Recommended Dosage
Calcium acetate	Tablet: 667 mg Gelcap: 667 mg	two tablets or gelcaps three times daily with meals
Calcium carbonate	Tablet, capsule, liquid, and powder; various strengths	1–2 g three times daily with meals
Aluminum hydroxide	Tablets: 300 and 600 mg Suspension: 320 mg/5 mL	1–2 tablets or 15–30 mL three or four times daily with meals and at bedtime

Source: From reference 42.

Table 6.6 **Treatment of Hypocalcemia**

Degree of Hypocalcemia	Preferred Calcium Salt	Intermittent Bolus Dosage	Continuous Infusion Dosage
Mild to moderate, asymptomatic	Gluconate	1–2 g calcium gluconate over 30–60 minutes; may repeat every 6 hours as needed	4.56–9.12 mEq calcium over 30–60 minutes; may repeat every 6 hours as needed
Severe, symptomatic	Chloride or gluconate	1,000 mg calcium chloride or 3 g calcium gluconate over 10 minutes; may repeat as needed	13.6 mEq calcium over 10 minutes; may repeat as needed

Source: From reference 42.

directions as a result of compensation. The compensation for metabolic alkalosis is a decrease in ventilation and increase in arterial $PaCO_2$. The compensation for metabolic acidosis is an increase in ventilation with a decrease in arterial $PaCO_2$. Two formulas are necessary to assess for complex acid-base disorders:

$$\text{Expected } PaCO_2 = (0.9 \times HCO_3^-) + 15$$
$$\text{Expected } HCO_3^- = (0.2 \times \Delta PaCO_2)$$

If the value is different from what is expected, a complex disorder is present.

The next step in analysis of a metabolic acidosis is to find a possible anion gap:

$$\text{anion gap} = [Na+] - ([Cl-] + [HCO3-])$$

An elevated anion gap acidosis is caused by ketones, uremia, lactate, or toxin (KULT). A known diagnostic error in calculating the anion gap can occur if the plasma chloride has increased due to recent administration of a colloid or a crystalloid. This results in iatrogenic hyperchloremia and a falsely increased anion gap. On the other hand, the anion gap might be falsely low, with decreased serum albumin but these are several unusual causes (Table 6.7).

Table 6.7 **Acid-Base Disorders**

Acid-Base Abnormality	pH	PaCO$_2$	HCO$_3^-$
Metabolic acidosis	↓	↓*	↓
Metabolic alkalosis	↑	↑*	↑
Respiratory alkalosis	↑	↓	~**
Respiratory acidosis	↓	↑	~**

* PaCO$_2$ too low respiratory alkalosis (less than 4 mm Hg from calculated value)
PaCO$_2$ too high respiratory acidosis (more than 4 mm Hg from calculated value)

** HCO$_3^-$ too low metabolic acidosis (less than 2 mEq/L from calculated value)
HCO$_3^-$ too high metabolic alkalosis (more than 2 mEq/L from calculated value)

Treatment of metabolic acidosis requires identification of etiology and only requires correction if the patient is severely acidotic. Serum sodium bicarbonate is used to control metabolic acidosis with the arterial pH < 7.0.[34,35] Metabolic alkalosis should be treated with extra saline or with acetazolamide if diuresis remains necessary. Other replacement therapies include potassium replacement in any hypokalemia, and management of diabetic ketoacidosis or nonketotic hyperglycemia.[1,16,18,26]

The treatment of respiratory acidosis is mechanical ventilation or bronchodilator therapy. Naloxone for opiate-induced hypoventilation and respiratory acidosis may be needed. The treatment of respiratory alkalosis may be simply adjusting the ventilator to decreased tidal volume and respiratory rate or sedation to control the ventilator driver. The main causes of acid-base disturbances in acutely ill neurologic patients are shown in Table 6.8.

Table 6.8 **Acid-Base Disorders**

Metabolic	
Acidosis	*Alkalosis*
Lactic acidosis, ketoacidosis	Contraction alkalosis
Renal failure	Parenteral nutrition
Intoxications	Bicarbonate therapy
Diarrhea	Corticosteroids
Respiratory	
Acidosis	*Alkalosis*
Pulmonary disease	Hyperventilation (central)
Narcotics	Anxiety
Upper airway obstruction	Fever
Inadequate ventilation	Hypoxemia
	Pulmonary disease

By the Way

Sodium Content and Osmolality in
Intravenous Fluid Solutions

Intravenous Fluid	Sodium Content (mmol per liter)	Osmolality
5% dextrose	0	252
0.45% sodium chloride	77	406
Lactated Ringer's	130	275
Albumin 5%	130	309
0.9% sodium chloride	154	308
1.5% sodium chloride	256	450
3% sodium chloride	513	900

Source: From reference 46.

Fluids and Electrolytes by the Numbers

- ~80% of acid-base disorders are mixed disorders
- ~60% of patients with SAH develop cerebral salt wasting
- ~50% of patients with acute brain injury are markedly dehydrated
- ~15% of patients with TBI develop diabetes insipidus
- ~10% of patients with acute brain injury develop hyponatremia

Putting It All Together

- Most neurologic patients require normal saline infusion
- Both hyponatremia and hypernatremia are common after acute brain injury and require adjustment of infusate
- Hypokalemia is ubiquitous in hospitalized patients. Often nasogastric suctioning is implicated
- Hypomagnesemia is related to drug administration, most often diuretics or antibiotics
- Hypophosphatemia can be a result of refeeding syndrome or insulin administration
- Anion gap calculation is needed to find the cause of metabolic acidosis

References

1. Agarwal A, Wingo CS. Treatment of hypokalemia. *N Engl J Med* 1999;340:154–155.
2. Agus ZS. Hypomagnesemia. *J Am Soc Nephrol* 1999;10:1616.
3. Aiyagari V, Deibert E, Diringer MN. Hypernatremia in the neurologic intensive care unit: how high is too high? *J Crit Care* 2006;21:163–172.
4. Al-Ghamdi SM, Cameron EC, Sutton RA. Magnesium deficiency: pathophysiologic and clinical overview. *Is J Kidney Dis* 1994;24:737–752.
5. Adrogue HJ, Madias NE. Hypernatremia. *N Engl J Med* 2000;342:1493–1499.
6. Adrogue HJ, Madias NE. Hyponatremia. *N Engl J Med* 2000;342:1581–1589.
7. Arora SK. Hypernatremic disorders in the intensive care unit. *J Intensive Care Med* 2013;28:37–45.
8. Berl T. Treating hyponatremia: damned if we do and damned if we don't. *Kidney Int* 1990;37:1006–1018.
9. Brochard L, Abroug F, Brenner M, et al. An official ATS/ERS/ESICM/SCCM/SRLF statement: prevention and management of acute renal failure in the ICU patient: an international consensus conference in intensive care medicine. *Am J Respir Crit Care Med* 2010;181:1128–1155.
10. Bushinsky DA, Monk RD. Calcium. *Lancet* 1998;352:306–311.
11. Chung HM, Kluge R, Schrier RW, Anderson RJ. Clinical assessment of extracellular fluid volume in hyponatremia. *Am J Med* 1987;83:905–908.
12. Clayton JA, Le Jeune IR, Hall IP. Severe hyponatremia in medical in-patients: etiology, assessment and outcome. *QJM* 2006;99:505–511.
13. Curry N, Davis PW. What's new in resuscitation strategies for the patient with multiple trauma? *Injury* 2012;43:1021–1028.
14. Dickerson RN, Brown RO. Hypomagnesemia in hospitalized patients receiving nutritional support. *Heart Lung* 1985;14:561–569.
15. Finfer S, Bellomo R, Boyce N, et al. A comparison of albumin and saline for fluid resuscitation in the intensive care unit. *N Engl J Med* 2004;350:2247–2256.
16. Freedman BI, Burkart JM. Hypokalemia. *Crit Care Clin* 1991;7:143–153.
17. Friedler RM, Koffler A, Kurokawa K. Hyponatremia and hypernatremia. *Clin Nephrol* 1977;7:163–172.
18. Gennari FJ. Hypokalemia. *N Engl J Med* 1998;339:451–458.
19. Hadjizacharia P, Beale EO, Inaba K, Chan LS, Demetriades D. Acute diabetes insipidus in severe head injury: a prospective study. *J Am Coll Surg* 2008;207:477–484.
20. Halevy J, Bulvik S. Severe hypophosphatemia in hospitalized patients. *Arch Intern Med* 1988;148:153–155.
21. Halperin ML, Bohn D. Clinical approach to disorders of salt and water balance: emphasis on integrative physiology. *Crit Care Clin* 2002;18:249–272.
22. Halperin ML, Kamel KS. Potassium. *Lancet* 1998;352:135–140.
23. Hoorn EJ, Halperin ML, Zietse R. Diagnostic approach to a patient with hyponatremia: traditional versus physiology-based options. *QJM* 2005;98:529–540.
24. Knochel JP. The pathophysiology and clinical characteristics of severe hypophosphatemia. *Arch Intern Med* 1977;137:203–220.
25. Kraft MD, Btaiche IF, Sacks GS, Kudsk KA. Treatment of electrolyte disorders in adult patients in the intensive care unit. *Am J Health Syst Pharm* 2005;62:1663–1682.
26. Kruse JA, Carlson RW. Rapid correction of hypokalemia using concentrated intravenous potassium chloride infusions. *Arch Intern Med* 1990;150:613–617.
27. Kumar S, Berl T. Sodium. *Lancet* 1998;352:220–228.
28. Laxenaire MC, Charpentier C, Feldman L. Anaphylactoid reactions to colloid plasma substitutes: incidence, risk factors, mechanisms; a French multicenter prospective study. *Ann Fr Anesth Reanim* 1994;13:301–310.
29. Lentz RD, Brown DM, Kjellstrand CM. Treatment of severe hypophosphatemia. *Ann Intern Med* 1978;89:941–944.

30. Lindner G, Funk GC, Schwarz C, et al. Hypernatremia in the critically ill is an independent risk factor for mortality. *Am J Kidney Dis* 2007;50:952–957.

31. Lindner G, Kneidinger N, Holzinger U, Druml W, Schwarz C. Tonicity balance in patients with hypernatremia acquired in the intensive care unit. *Am J Kidney Dis* 2009;54:674–679.

32. McManus ML, Churchwell KB, Strange K. Regulation of cell volume in health and disease. *N Engl J Med* 1995;333:1260–1266.

33. Moritz ML, Ayus JC. Hospital-acquired hyponatremia—why are hypotonic parenteral fluids still being used? *Nat Clin Pract Nephrol* 2007;3:374–382.

34. Morris CG, Low J. Metabolic acidosis in the critically ill: part 1. Classification and pathophysiology. *Anaesthesia* 2008;63:294–301.

35. Morris CG, Low J. Metabolic acidosis in the critically ill: part 2. Causes and treatment. *Anaesthesia* 2008;63:396–411.

36. Myburgh J, Cooper DJ, Finfer S, et al. Saline or albumin for fluid resuscitation in patients with traumatic brain injury. *N Engl J Med* 2007;357:874–884.

37. Nguyen MK, Kurtz I. New insights into the pathophysiology of the dysnatremias: a quantitative analysis. *Am J Physiol Renal Physiol* 2004;287:F172–F180.

38. Reinhart K, Perner A, Sprung CL, et al. Consensus statement of the ESICM task force on colloid volume therapy in critically ill patients. *Intensive Care Med* 2012;38:368–383.

39. Reinhart RA, Desbiens NA. Hypomagnesemia in patients entering the ICU. *Crit Care Med* 1985;13:506–507.

40. Ring J, Messmer K. Incidence and severity of anaphylactoid reactions to colloid volume substitutes. *Lancet* 1977;1:466–469.

41. Ritz E. Acute hypophosphatemia. *Kidney Int* 1982;22:84–94.

42. Rose BD, Post TW. *Clinical Physiology of Acid-Base and Electrolyte Disorders* 5th ed. New York, McGraw-Hill, 2001, 441.

43. Schneider AG, Baldwin I, Freitag E, Glassford N, Bellomo R. Estimation of fluid status changes in critically ill patients: Fluid balance chart or electronic bed weight? *J Crit Care* 2012;27(745):e7–e12.

44. Sedlacek M, Schoolwerth AC, Remillard BD. Electrolyte disturbances in the intensive care unit. *Semin Dial* 2006;19:496–501.

45. Sterns RH, Hix JK, Silver SM. Management of hyponatremia in the ICU. *Chest* 2013; 144:672–679.

46. Wijdicks EFM, Rabinstein AA. *Neurocritical Care*. New York, Oxford University Press, 2011.

47. Williams ME. Hyperkalemia. *Crit Care Clin* 1991;7:155–174.

48. Yee AH, Burns JD, Wijdicks EFM. Cerebral salt wasting: pathophysiology, diagnosis, and treatment. *Neurosurg Clin N Am* 2010;21:339–352.

7

Glucose Adjustment

Susceptibility to hyperglycemia—rising or fluctuating serum glucose—is common in patients with acute brain injury, but also in any acute medical condition that incites a major stress response. Alteration of the carbohydrate metabolism can be expected in acute illness, and in the past this response was called "stress diabetes."[69] This was not surprising to clinicians, who felt that under the circumstances this was a normal physiologic event—a more severe "stress response" in more severe brain injuries. It was also not surprising that it could lead to a poor outcome.[40,42,55]

When studies in cardiac surgery—in the early 2000s—found that aggressive control of diabetes with insulin therapy could decrease wound infections and also improve outcome, the approach to hyperglycemia changed.[22] The larger idea was that acute hyperglycemia could be harmful to the patient. It became even more urgent when randomized clinical trials from Leuven found that aggressive hyperglycemia control in nondiabetic patients with medical or surgical critical illness could improve outcome.[66,67] This spurred tight glucose control for any sick patient, including neurologic patients.[57]

The results of the—definitive—NICE-SUGAR clinical trial published in 2009, found that strict glucose control to 81–108 mg/dL (4.5 to 6.0 mmol/L) could lead to worse outcomes.[47] That finding brought a halt to very tight management of blood glucose. Furthermore, a subsequent study (SPECS) found that strict glucose control in children undergoing cardiac surgery did not improve outcomes by any outcome measure.[1] It is now quite clear that claims of improved outcomes with intense control of serum glucose in the general critically ill population are exaggerated at best and at worst are simply untrue.

A concerning hyperglycemia is mostly understood as a serum glucose concentration of more than 120 mg/dL (or 7 mmol/L). Far more relevant in view of this is how an injured brain fares with different levels of hyperglycemia. How does the brain handle changes in blood glucose? How aggressively do we have to lower the blood glucose, and what are the risks of hypoglycemia? Is sustained hyperglycemia worse for the brain than brief hypoglycemia? How reliable is bedside (point-of-care) testing of glucose? How does the vast body of qualitatively diverse literature pertain to the clinical practice of treating acute neurologic patients? This chapter provides answers to these common questions and describes the best approach knowing what we know now.

Principles

Glucose demand in the brain is generally high and relates to the degree of neuro-nal activity—as expected the need is highest in the cortex. Already under basal conditions the brain consumes 80% of glucose availability. Uptake of glucose in the brain does not require insulin but is brought in through glucose transporters. There are central and peripheral specialized neurons (glucosensors) that increase their activity when blood sugar rises.[72]

How is the brain linked to glucose control? There is a coordinated multipathway response. Peripheral sensors in the portal mesenteric vein and small intestines signal to the hypothalamus and solitary nucleus mostly through the vagus nerve X. The vagal nerve efferents into the pancreas increase the secretion of insulin and reduce catecholamines. Simultaneously, neurons in the ventromedial hypothalamus release an inhibitory (sympathetic) action on the pancreas that results in insulin production to lower hyperglycemia (Figure 7.1).

Hypoglycemia results in increased firing of the nucleus tractus solitarius and the lateral hypothalamic glucose sensors. This decreases parasympathetic

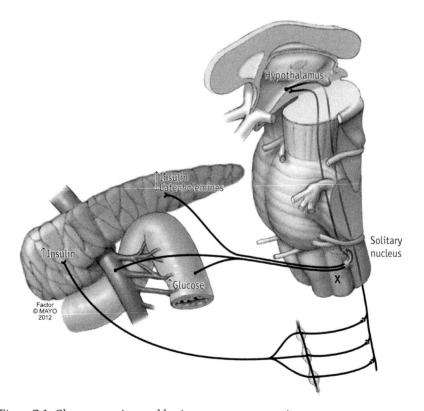

Figure 7.1 Glucose sensing and brain-pancreas connection.

activity, increases sympathetic outflow through the lateral hypothalamus, and elevates blood glucose level by promoting glycogenolysis and reduction of insulin secretion.[72] Recurrent hypoglycemia (as in type 1 diabetes mellitus) may cause a reduced counterregulation (much lower levels of hypoglycemia are needed to produce a response).[3]

How does hyperglycemia occur? Patients who have become acutely ill may be in so-called hypermetabolic state. This state is associated with increasing counterregulatory hormone responses. There is peripheral insulin resistance and increase in hepatic glucose production. Hyperglycemia is promoted by hepatic glycogenolysis as a result of increased catecholamines and as a result of sympathetic stimulation of glycogen breakdown. Patients who are hypermetabolic also have dramatic increase in glucagon levels, but with insulin concentration increased to a lesser extent.[25] Furthermore, if there is significant injury to the body due to trauma or other stressor, an insulin-resistant state may occur in which hyperglycemia occurs despite normal or increased plasma insulin concentration.[49] Plasma cortisol is elevated and potentiates the action of glucagon and epinephrine on the liver. Stress hyperglycemia can also be caused by administration of a large amount of glucose (for example, during parenteral nutrition) but also by D5W (5% dextrose in water) and lactated Ringer's bolus infusions.

Glucose uptake by carriers such as GLUT-4 may also be diminished. Generally, increased level of cytokines, glucagon, cortisol growth hormone, and catecholamines upregulate the hepatic glucose production.[51,60] These factors may also oppose the normal insulin action and increase lipolysis and proteinolysis, which are fuel substrates for gluconeogenesis.

Hyperglycemia has a combination of effects. First, osmotic diuresis with hypovolemia may occur. Second, hyperglycemia has been linked to oxidative stress, increased excitotoxicity, increase in tissue lactate, and even increased likelihood of thrombosis, causing changes in brain circulation at a micro level.[26,29] The effects of hyperglycemia are well known and summarized in Figure 7.2.[4,44]

How does hyperglycemia injure brain or worsen brain injury? After brain injury there is an increase in cerebral metabolism from hyperglycolysis.[5] There is an increase in anaerobic metabolism, and metabolic demand might be further increased by seizures. Limiting the availability of the brain's major substrate could potentially lead to further injury. Hyperglycemia may increase lactate levels (Figure 7.3) and acidosis may exacerbate neuronal injury, particularly in the penumbral zone through free radical formation, glutamate release with, eventually, abnormal intracellular calcium regulation, and mitochondrial failure.[37] On a microscopic level, hyperglycemia may impair astrocyte reactivity, and may increase neuronal and glial apoptosis, particularly in the hippocampus and frontal cortex. Microglial activation in hyperglycemia may induce inflammatory cytokine production, and is demonstrated a few days after sustained hyperglycemia. The general understanding is that hyperglycemia increases oxidative

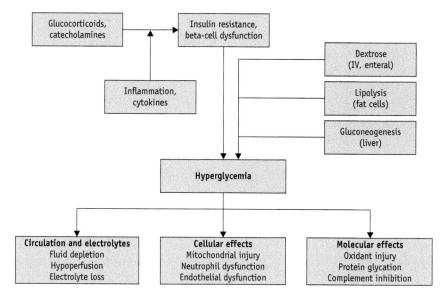

Figure 7.2 The effects of hyperglycemia.

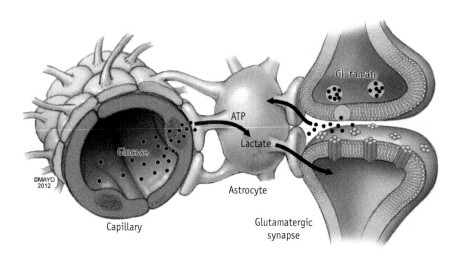

Figure 7.3 Glucose in neurons. The astrocyte takes up glutamate from the synaptic cleft and its recycling results in a decline in ATP. This will result in GLUT transport pores to open and glucose enters the astrocyte and is converted into lactate used by the neuron. (From Peters et al. Am J Hum Biol 2011;2329–2334.)

stress at the cellular level, which then activates enzymatic pathways of glucose metabolism that may eventually develop neuronal damage.[17,27,64]

However, there is more to it. During aerobic metabolism, glucose normally produces 38 moles of adenosine triphosphate (ATP) per mole of glucose. This is very energy efficient. In an ischemic brain, glucose is metabolized anaerobically and produces lactate and only 2 moles of ATP per mole of glucose. The ATP is hydrolyzed during consumption, producing hydrogen ions that with lactate cause lactic acidosis. Acidosis in neurons impairs ion hemostasis. More glucose, more hydrogen ions, more lactate, more acidosis. This is also known as the "glucose paradox of ischemia." In ischemic stroke, reperfusion may also worsen tissue acidosis (but only if reperfusion occurs). The damage occurs regardless of the cause of hyperglycemia, and the effect—in animal experiments—exists even with hyperglycemia after the injury.

Experimental studies have found that infusion of glucose-containing solutions before global and focal ischemic results in significant worsening of postischemic outcome.[2] In ischemic stroke it also has become apparent that hyperglycemia with its associated excess lactate production becomes "neurotoxic" and may convert a penumbra into infarction. Patients with hyperglycemia may also more rapidly develop cerebral infarction, which may nullify the effects of restoration of circulation. Patients with diabetes after an ischemic insult have a worse outcome than patients who have no diabetes.

Thus, in the end, insulin might have significant beneficial actions. It not only stimulates glucose uptake and energy production but also has an anti-inflammatory property and reduces oxygen radical formation. Insulin also suppresses the insulin-like growth factor, increases muscle protein synthesis, inhibits apoptosis, and promotes repair of damaged tissue and promotes ischemic reconditioning. Some studies have found that insulin results in less ischemia/reperfusion damage.

Hypoglycemia (unless prolonged) does not necessarily damage the brain.[58,63] Many diabetics have series of hypoglycemic attacks or even series of hypoglycemic comas without long-lasting effects. Nonetheless, one severe unrecognized hypoglycemic attack can cause persistent coma. Hypoglycemia in an already-injured astrocyte may cause further injury.[47] One study with aggressive brain glucose reduction found that intensively treated patients exhibited markers of cellular distress, showing increased oxygen extraction fraction and abnormal lactate/pyruvate ratio.[68] In critically ill patients, severe hypoglycemia (less than 40 mg/dL) increases the probability of death due to increased risk for vasodilatation and hypotension and cardiac arrhythmias. Infusion with insulin is also a strong risk factor for mortality if hypoglycemia occurs.[49]

Thus hypoglycemia damages the injured brain, and there is sufficient evidence that the threshold beyond which injury occurs has been lowered. A poorly perfused brain is also far more susceptible to a hypoglycemic insult.[58,59] The serum glucose level may not be a good marker of brain glucose, and some studies have suggested that glucose levels within the normal range (80–100 mg/dL) may already cause increased glucose utilization by the brain.

In Practice

The debate regarding intensive versus standard glucose management has been resolved with the findings of the 2009 NICE-SUGAR trial, and protocols for glucose management in critically ill patients are well established.[15,23] Control of hyperglycemia using sliding-scale insulin regimes or infusion followed by sub-cutaneous insulin did reduce infection rate in a systemic review.[30,45] Control of hyperglycemia may also reduce critical illness polyneuropathy.[65]

There are questions about safety and efficacy of insulin therapy in critically ill neurologic and neurosurgical patients.[7,9,10,21,50,62] Only a few small randomized trials have been performed in neurocritically ill patients.[6,13,24] The best glucose target remains to be further determined, and in all fairness is nothing more than a "guesstimate."[20,41,53,73] The most current data is summarized in Table 7.1.

For the practitioner (and nursing staff closely involved with titration of glu-cose infusions), the recommendations lack uniformity (Table 7.2). Currently, the American Association of Clinical Endocrinologists and the American Diabetic Association define best practice for inpatient glucose control as initiation of continuous intravenous insulin at a threshold not higher than 180 mg/dL with a blood glucose target between 140 and 180 mg/dL. A blood glucose of <110 mg/dL is not considered safe.

Frequent hypoglycemic episodes can lead to a "yo-yo effect" that may be interpreted as glycemic variability. Blood glucose rebounds after

Table 7.1 **Acute Brain Injury and Glucose: The Evidence**

Ischemic stroke	• Glucose administration 110–126 mg/dL increased mortality[11]
	• Glucose ≥155 mg/dL increased poor outcome[16]
Cerebral hemorrhage	• Increase of 18 mg/dL increased mortality
	• Glucose ≥164 mg/dL increased mortality[19]
	• Hematoma expansion reduced with glucose control[53]
Subarachnoid hemorrhage	• Any hyperglycemia increases in-hospital complications and poor outcome
Traumatic brain injury	• Hyperglycemia >200 mg/dL increases mortality[24]
Anoxic-ischemic injury after cardiac arrest	• Low probability of awakening[39]

Table 7.2 **Current Recommendations for Glycemic Control in Critically Ill Patients**

Organization	Year	Patient Population	Treatment Threshold (mg/dL)	Target Glucose Level (mg/dL)
Canadian Diabetes Association	2008	ICU	110	80–110
American Heart Association	2008	CCU	180	90–140
Society of Thoracic Surgeons	2009	SICU	150	<150
European Society of Cardiology	2009	SICU	180	140–180
Surviving Sepsis Campaign	2009	ICU	180	<150
Institute for Healthcare Improvement	2009	ICU	180	<180
American Diabetes Association	2011	ICU	180	140–180
American College of Physicians	2011	ICU	180	140–180

ICU = intensive care unit; CCU = coronary care unit; SICU = surgical intensive care unit

administration of dextrose and vice versa declines with use of insulin causing marked variability—a clinical observation that has been associated with poor outcome.

In practice it is important to follow serum glucose from admission and start an insulin sliding scale or insulin infusion. Optimal glucose control on the ward or in an intensive care unit can be achieved with current hospital laboratory systems, and point-of-care devices may be quite helpful. Unfortunately these bedside "point-of-care" glucose meters—when reading from a capillary finger stick—tend to systematically overestimate the blood glucose value.[14,32] Falsely elevated glucose results may lead to improper insulin administration and increase the risk of hypoglycemia. Therefore, a reflex response to hyperglycemia may be detrimental to the patient—repeating tests and refraining from changing insulin dosing until a trend is observed is more appropriate. Degree of inaccuracy of these devices has remained in the order of 20%. Glucose levels from an arterial line or central venous catheter are more reliable. The alternative—delays using a central laboratory, multiple phlebotomies, and blood loss associated with frequent punctures—justifies multiple point-of-care glucose measurements.

In patients with acute neurologic injury, the question is whether avoidance of hyperglycemia in the first 3 days of symptom onset is the most optimal approach. Some studies have found that hyperglycemia on admission was not associated with worse outcome, but persistent hyperglycemia worsened outcome and ischemic stroke.[19,28,31,34,36,52,54,61,69,70]

There is no consistent data that proves insulin-infusion protocols impact outcome in neurologic patients, and several studies have reported high percentages of hypoglycemia with strict control (defined as less than 120 mg/dL).[8,35,38] The costs and workload of insulin protocols and possible harmful effects when stricter control is implemented are concerns and may become barriers to using these protocols.[33,43,56]

An example of an insulin sliding scale is shown in Table 7.3. One should obtain preprandial glucose values except in patients with continuous nasogastric feeding. Patients with bolus feedings are not eligible, nor are patients with a ketoacidosis, which requires a different approach and a consult by endocrinology. The insulin infusion can be discontinued when the insulin infusion has been stopped for 4 hours. Aggressive glucose control is also discontinued after the patient has made a substantial improvement. Glucose point-of-care testing can be continued at 6-hour intervals and for 2 days after the infusion has been stopped.

In some patients a marked hyperglycemia is found; values can approach 800–1,000 mg/dL. This may indicate a previously undiagnosed hyperosmolar hyperglycemic state (HHS) or diabetic ketoacidosis (DKA). Laboratory evaluation can differentiate these two conditions quickly with serum glucose (much higher in

Table 7.3 **Protocol for IV Insulin Infusion in patients with hyperglycemia**

- 250 units of Novolin R insulin in 250 mL of 0.45% sodium chloride (1 unit/mL)
- Monitor glucose POC levels every hour.
- Infuse insulin into existing line of compatible IV solution.
- If blood glucose remains above 150 mg/dL and does not decrease, increase the baseline infusion rate by 2 units per hour.
- Target blood glucose: 140–180 mg/dL (usually less than 150 mg/dL)

Glucose POC (mg/dL)	Insulin Infusion Rate (units/h)
>400	16
351 – 400	14
301 – 350	12
251 – 300	10
201 – 250	8
171 – 200	5
151 – 170	3
131 – 150	2
111 – 130	1
60 – 110	0

POC: Point of Care

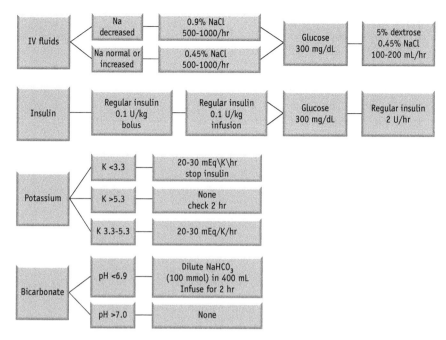

Figure 7.4 Treatment of hyperglycemic emergencies.

HHS), arterial blood gas (metabolic acidosis with DKA), urine ketones (DKA), or serum osmolality (increased in HHS). HbA1C is elevated in any poorly controlled or undiagnosed diabetes and is normal in a stress response.

The treatment of both these conditions has some similarities, but also major differences in management. These are foremost: fluid administration to rehydrate (up to 5 liters administration in DKA and up to 10 liters in HHS), type of fluid (normal saline—with hypernatremia or half-normal isotonic saline with nor-monatremia), hydration rate (usually 500 mL per hour), potassium supplementation (20–40 mEq with K between 3.3 and 5.3) and, in DKA, use of bicarbonate with pH less than 6.9. This chapter is not the place for an in depth discussion of acute hyperglycemia, but suggestions for acute treatment are shown in Figure 7.4.

Putting It All Together

- There is a complex glucose sensor system that corrects fluctuations
- Hyperglycemia damages the brain through worsening lactic acidosis
- Normal serum glucose levels may already cause increased glucose utilization by the brain
- Control hyperglycemia, but maintain at least values between 140–180 mg/dL
- Point-of-care testing remains useful but may overestimates glucose values

---

By the Way

- The amount of blood impacts capillary blood glucose measurements
- Low hematocrit may result in high glucose levels
- Poor peripheral perfusion may change point-of-care results
- Drugs may interfere with glucose measurements (e.g., levodopa, dopamine, mannitol, acetaminophen)
- Postprandial glucose (2 hours after meal) may lead to overuse of insulin

---

Glucose by the Numbers

- ~80% of patients with traumatic brain injury develop hyperglycemia
- ~40% of patients with a stroke have hyperglycemia and no diabetes
- ~30% increased risk of mortality if hyperglycemic after cerebral hematoma
- ~15% of patients develop hypoglycemia with intense glucose control
- ~5% reduced mortality with glucose control after traumatic brain injury

---

References

1. Agus MSD, Steil GM, Pywij D, et al. Tight glycemic control versus standard care after pediatric cardiac surgery. *N Engl J Med* 2012;367:1208–1209.
2. Baird TA, Parsons MW, Phanh T, et al. Persistent poststroke hyperglycemia is independently associated with infarct expansion and worse clinical outcome. *Stroke* 2003;34:2208–2214.
3. Beall C, Ashford ML, McCrimmon RJ. The physiology and pathophysiology of the neural control of the counterregulatory response. *Am J Physiol Regul Integr Comp Physiol* 2012;302:R215–223.
4. Benarroch EE. Glycogen metabolism: metabolic coupling between astrocytes and neurons. *Neurology* 2010;74:919–923.
5. Bergsneider M, Hovda DA, Shalmon E, et al. Cerebral hyperglycolysis following severe traumatic brain injury in humans: a positron emission tomography study. *J Neurosurg* 199;86:241–251.
6. Bilotta F, Caramia R, Cernak I, et al. Intensive insulin therapy after severe traumatic brain injury: a randomized clinical trial. *Neurocrit Care* 2008;9:159–166.
7. Bilotta F, Caramia R, Paoloni FP, et al. Safety and efficacy of intensive insulin therapy in critical neurosurgical patients. *Anesthesiology* 2009;110:611–619.
8. Bilotta F, Giovannini F, Caramia R, Rosa G. Glycemia management in neurocritical care patients: a review. *J Neurosurg Anesthesiol* 2009;21:2–9.
9. Bilotta F, Spinelli A, Giovannini F, et al. The effect of intensive insulin therapy on infection rate, vasospasm, neurologic outcome, and mortality in neurointensive care unit after intracranial aneurysm clipping in patients with acute subarachnoid hemorrhage: a randomized prospective pilot trial. *J Neurosurg Anesthesiol* 2007;19:156–160.

10. Bruno A, Kent TA, Coull BM, et al. Treatment of hyperglycemia in ischemic stroke (THIS): a randomized pilot trial. *Stroke* 2008;39:384–389.
11. Capes SE, Hunt D, Malmberg K, et al. Stress hyperglycemia and prognosis of stroke in non-diabetic and diabetic patients: a systematic overview. *Stroke* 2001;32:2426–2432.
12. Cely CM, Arora P, Quartin AA, et al. Relationship of baseline glucose homeostasis to hyperglycemia during medical critical illness. *Chest* 2004;126:879–887.
13. Coester A, Neumann CR, Schmidt MI. Intensive insulin therapy in severe traumatic brain injury: a randomized trial. *J Trauma* 2010;68:904–911.
14. Critchell CD, Savarese V, Callahan A, et al. Accuracy of bedside capillary blood glucose measurements in critically ill patients. *Intensive Care Med* 2007;33:2079–2084.
15. Egi M, Finfer S, Bellomo R. Glycemic control in the ICU. *Chest* 2011;140:212–220.
16. Fuentes B, Castillo J, San Jose B, et al. The prognostic value of capillary glucose levels in acute stroke: the GLycemia in Acute Stroke (GLIAS) study. *Stroke* 2009;40:562–568.
17. Garg R, Chaudhuri A, Munschauer F, Dandona P. Hyperglycemia, insulin, and acute ischemic stroke: a mechanistic justification for a trial of insulin infusion therapy. *Stroke* 2006;37:267–273.
18. Godoy DA, Di Napoli M, Rabinstein AA. Treating hyperglycemia in neurocritical patients: benefits and perils. *Neurocrit Care* 2010;13:425–438.
19. Godoy DA, Piñero GR, Svampa S, et al. Hyperglycemia and short-term outcome in patients with spontaneous intracerebral hemorrhage. *Neurocrit Care* 2008;9:217–229.
20. Gray CS, Hildreth AJ, Sandercock PA, et al. Glucose-potassium-insulin infusions in the management of post-stroke hyperglycaemia: the UK Glucose Insulin in Stroke Trial (GIST-UK). *Lancet Neurol* 2007;6:397–406.
21. Green DM, O'Phelan KH, Bassin SL, et al. Intensive versus conventional insulin therapy in critically ill neurologic patients. *Neurocrit Care* 2010;13:299–306.
22. Grey NJ, Perdrizet GA. Reduction of nosocomial infections in the surgical intensive-care unit by strict glycemic control. *Endocr Pract* 2004;10 Suppl 2:46–52.
23. Griesdale DE, de Souza RJ, van Dam RM, et al. Intensive insulin therapy and mortality among critically ill patients: a meta-analysis including NICE-SUGAR study data. *CMAJ* 2009;180:821–827.
24. Griesdale DE, Tremblay MH, McEwen J, Chittock DR. Glucose control and mortality in patients with severe traumatic brain injury. *Neurocrit Care* 2009;11:311–316.
25. Gruetter R. Glycogen: the forgotten cerebral energy store. *J Neurosci Res* 2003;74:179–183.
26. Hutchinson PJ, O'Connell MT, Seal A, et al. A combined microdialysis and FDG-PET study of glucose metabolism in head injury. *Acta Neurochir* 2009;151:51–61.
27. Jacka MJ, Torok-Both CJ, Bagshaw SM. Blood glucose control among critically ill patients with brain injury. *Can J Neurol Sci* 2009;36:436–442.
28. Jeremitsky E, Omert LA, Dunham CM, et al. The impact of hyperglycemia on patients with severe brain injury. *J Trauma* 2005;58:47–50.
29. Jeschke MG, Klein D, Bolder U, Einspanier R. Insulin attenuates the systemic inflammatory response in endotoxemic rats. *Endocrinology* 2004;145:4084–4093.
30. Jeschke MG, Klein D, Herndon DN. Insulin treatment improves the systemic inflammatory reaction to severe trauma. *Ann Surg* 2004;239:553–560.
31. Johnston KC, Hall CE, Kissela BM, et al. Glucose regulation in acute stroke patients (GRASP) trial: a randomized pilot trial. *Stroke* 2009;40:3804–3809.
32. Kanji S, Buffie J, Hutton B, et al. Reliability of point-of-care testing for glucose measurement in critically ill adults. *Crit Care Med* 2005;33:2778–2785.
33. Kansagara D, Fu R, Freeman M, Wolf F, Helfand M. Intensive insulin therapy in hospitalized patients: a systematic review. *Ann Intern Med* 2011;154:268–282.
34. Kimura K, Iguchi Y, Inoue T, et al. Hyperglycemia independently increases the risk of early death in acute spontaneous intracerebral hemorrhage. *J Neurol Sci* 2007;255:90–94.
35. Kruyt ND, Biessels GJ, de Haan RJ, et al. Hyperglycemia and clinical outcome in aneurysmal subarachnoid hemorrhage: a meta-analysis. *Stroke* 2009;40:e424–e430.
36. Kruyt ND, Biessels GJ, Devries JH, Roos YB. Hyperglycemia in acute ischemic stroke: pathophysiology and clinical management. *Nat Rev Neurol* 2010;6:145–155.

37. Li PA, Shuaib A, Miyashita H, et al. Hyperglycemia enhances extracellular glutamate accumulation in rats subjected to forebrain ischemia. *Stroke* 2000;31:183–192.

38. Lingsma HF, Roozenbeek B, Steyerberg EW, et al. Early prognosis in traumatic brain injury: from prophecies to predictions. *Lancet Neurol* 2010;9:543–554.

39. Longstreth WT Jr, Inui TS. High blood glucose level on hospital admission and poor neurological recovery after cardiac arrest. *Ann Neurol* 1984;15:59–63.

40. Margulies DR, Hiatt JR, Vinson D Jr, Shabot MM. Relationship of hyperglycemia and severity of illness to neurologic outcome in head injury patients. *Am Surg* 1994;60:387–390.

41. Marik PE, Varon J. Intensive insulin therapy in the ICU: is it now time to jump off the bandwagon? *Resuscitation* 2007;74:191–193.

42. Marik PE, Bellomo R. Stress hyperglycemia: an essential survival response! *Crit Care* 2013;17(2):305.

43. McCormick MT, Muir KW, Gray CS, Walters MR. Management of hyperglycemia in acute stroke: how, when, and for whom? *Stroke* 2008;39:2177–2185.

44. Mizock BA. Alterations in fuel metabolism in critical illness: hyperglycaemia. *Best Pract Res Clin Endocrinol Metab* 2001;15:533–551.

45. Murad MH, Coburn JA, Coto-Yglesias F, et al. Glycemic control in non-critically ill hospitalized patients: a systematic review and meta-analysis. *J Clin Endocrinol Metab* 2012;97:49–58.

46. Murray GD, Butcher I, McHugh GS, et al. Multivariable prognostic analysis in traumatic brain injury: results from the IMPACT study. *J Neurotrauma* 2007;24:329–337.

47. Musen G, Simonson DC, Driscoll A et al. Regional brain activation during hypoglycemia in type 1 diabetes. *J Clin Endocrinol Metab* 2008;93:1450–1457.

48. NICE-SUGAR Study Investigators, Finfer S, Chittock DR, et al. Intensive versus conventional glucose control in critically ill patients. *N Engl J Med* 2009;360:1283–1297.

49. NICE-SUGAR Study Investigators, Finfer S, Liu B, et al. Hypoglycemia and risk of death in critically ill patients. *N Engl J Med* 2012;367:1108–1118.

50. Oddo M, Schmidt JM, Mayer SA, Chiolero RL. Glucose control after severe brain injury. *Curr Opin Clin Nutr Metab Care* 2008;11:134–139.

51. Oz G, Kumar A, Rao JP, et al. Human brain glycogen metabolism during and after hypoglycemia. *Diabetes* 2009;58:1978–1985.

52. Oz G, Seaquist ER, Kumar A, et al. Human brain glycogen content and metabolism: implications on its role in brain energy metabolism. *Am J Physiol Endocrinol Metab* 2007;292:E946–951.

53. Qureshi AI, Palesch YY, Martin R, et al. Association of serum glucose concentrations during acute hospitalization with hematoma expansion, perihematomal edema, and three month outcome among patients with intracerebral hemorrhage. *Neurocrit Care* 2011;15:428–435.

54. Radermecker RP, Scheen AJ. Management of blood glucose in patients with stroke. *Diabetes Metab* 2010;36 Suppl 3:S94–99.

55. Rovlias A, Kotsou S. The influence of hyperglycemia on neurological outcome in patients with severe head injury. *Neurosurgery* 2000;46:335–342;discussion 342–343.

56. Salim A, Hadjizacharia P, Dubose J, et al. Persistent hyperglycemia in severe traumatic brain injury: an independent predictor of outcome. *Am Surg* 2009;75:25–29.

57. Scurlock C, Raikhelkar J, Mechanick JI. The economics of glycemic control in the ICU in the United States. *Curr Opin Clin Nutr Metab Care* 2011;14:209–212.

58. Sieber FE, Derrer SA, Saudek CD, Traystman RJ. Effect of hypoglycemia on cerebral metabolism and carbon dioxide responsivity. *Am J Physiol* 1989;256:H697–H706.

59. Sieber FE, Koehler RC, Derrer SA, et al. Hypoglycemia and cerebral autoregulation in anesthetized dogs. *Am J Physiol* 1990;258:H1714–H1721.

60. Siesjo BK, Ingvar M, Pelligrino D. Regional differences in vascular autoregulation in the rat brain in severe insulin-induced hypoglycemia. *J Cereb Blood Flow Metab* 1983;3:478–485.

61. Simpson IA, Carruthers A, Vannucci SJ. Supply and demand in cerebral energy metabolism: the role of nutrient transporters. *J Cereb Blood Flow Metab* 2007;27:1766–1791.

62. Staszewski J, Brodacki B, Kotowicz J, et al. Intravenous insulin therapy in the maintenance of strict glycemic control in nondiabetic acute stroke patients with mild hyperglycemia. *J Stroke Cerebrovasc Dis* 2011;20:150–154.
63. Suh SW, Hamby AM, Swanson RA. Hypoglycemia, brain energetics, and hypoglycemic neuronal death. *Glia* 2007;55:1280–1286.
64. Timofeev I, Carpenter KL, Nortje J, et al. Cerebral extracellular chemistry and outcome following traumatic brain injury: a microdialysis study of 223 patients. *Brain* 2011;134:484–494.
65. Van den Berghe G, Schoonheydt K, Becx P, et al. Insulin therapy protects the central and peripheral nervous system of intensive care patients. *Neurology* 2005;64:1348–1353.
66. Van den Berghe G, Wilmer A, Hermans G, et al. Intensive insulin therapy in the medical ICU. *N Engl J Med* 2006;354:449–461.
67. Van den Berghe G, Wouters P, Weekers F, et al. Intensive insulin therapy in critically ill patients. *N Engl J Med* 2001;345:1359–1367.
68. Vespa P, Boonyaputthikul R, McArthur DL, et al. Intensive insulin therapy reduces microdialysis glucose values without altering glucose utilization or improving the lactate/pyruvate ratio after traumatic brain injury. *Crit Care Med* 2006;34:850–856.
69. Virkamäki A, Yki-Järvinen H. Mechanisms of insulin resistance during acute endotoxemia. *Endocrinology* 1994;134:2072–2078.
70. Vriesendorp TM, Roos YB, Kruyt ND, et al. Efficacy and safety of two 5 day insulin dosing regimens to achieve strict glycaemic control in patients with acute ischemic stroke. *J Neurol Neurosurg Psychiatry* 2009;80:1040–1043.
71. Walters MR, Weir CJ, Lees KR. A randomized, controlled pilot study to investigate the potential benefit of intervention with insulin in hyperglycemic acute ischemic stroke patients. *Cerebrovasc Dis* 2006;22:116–122.
72. Watts AG, Donovan CM. Sweet talk in the brain: glucosensing, neural networks, and hypoglycemic counterregulation. *Front Neuroendocrinol* 2010;31:32–43.
73. Wiener RS, Wiener DC, Larson RJ. Benefits and risks of tight glucose control in critically ill adults: a meta-analysis. *JAMA* 2008;300:933–944.
74. Yoder J. Tight glucose control after brain injury is unproven and unsafe. *J Neurosurg Anesthesiol* 2009;21:55–57.

8

Anticoagulation Strategies

Decisions on anticoagulation are often part of general care of acutely ill neurologic patients, and the how and the why come into play in three clinical situations.

First, although it has been established that immediate anticoagulant therapy in most patients with an acute stroke provides little short term benefits, when due to cardiogenic emboli heparin and warfarin could prevent reoccurrence. In cerebral venous thrombosis, immediate high-intensity heparinization or low molecular weight heparin is required.[43]

Second, there has been a significant increase in patients treated with warfarin and rapid reversal of its ongoing effect is needed when a patient presents with a cerebral hemorrhage. Reversal of anticoagulation could also involve reversal of intravenous heparin, and more recently the far more challenging thrombin inhibitors.[1,5] Reversal of warfarin is indicated even if there is a marginally increased international normalized ratio (INR), because any patient with a warfarin-associated intracranial hemorrhage is at risk of expansion of the hematoma. Expansion of the hematoma is common in the first hours, and trying to limit this unwanted progression has to be the major focus. In other patients, intracranial hemorrhage may be associated with a coagulopathy that needs attention, such as inherited disorders of platelet function, coagulopathy of liver dysfunction, other factor deficiencies or acute leukemia.

Third, as a consequence of immobilization, the risk of deep vein thrombosis (and pulmonary emboli) is increased. Unilateral hemiplegia (any acute hemispheric injury) or bilateral hemiplegia (acute spinal cord injury or Guillain-Barré syndrome) profoundly increases the risk of deep vein thrombosis and there is an obligation to institute aggressive preventive measures.[20]

In order to develop an anti coagulation strategy we need to answer a few questions. How do we best reverse anticoagulation, and how do we monitor its effect? What are the risks of restarting anticoagulation in a patient with a recent hemorrhage? How do we best prevent venous clots in an immobilized patient? This chapter provides the background of management of anticoagulation.

Principles

Some background is needed on how anticoagulation works and how it can be reversed. There are different drugs with different targets. The coagulation pathways and inhibiting drugs are shown in Figure 8.1. In this section we will provide some details.

SOME BASICS ON ANTICOAGULATION

Oral anticoagulants used throughout the world are usually warfarin or phenprocoumon. The two drugs are fairly comparable: Phenprocoumon has a longer half-life (up to 80 days), and the new steady state takes about 28 days as opposed to 7 days with warfarin. Phenprocoumon is also much more difficult to regulate, and reaching a therapeutic INR is two to three times longer than warfarin. Warfarin is used in the United States and thus discussed in more detail here.

A common approach is to start anticoagulation with IV heparin. Heparin binds with antithrombin III. This bind enhances its inhibiting activity—not only thrombin antifactor Xa, but also factors IXa, XIa, and XIIa.[39,40] Heparin causes a conformational change in antithrombin III, resulting in enhanced activation of antithrombin, quite significantly—more than 1,000-fold. There is a domino effect. Binding of factor Xa also reduces the conversion from prothrombin to thrombin, and diminished thrombin reduces the conversion change from fibrinogen to fibrin clot, as indicated in Figure 8.1. Low-molecular-weight

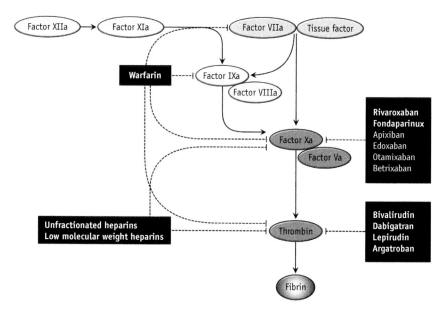

Figure 8.1 Targets of drugs on coagulation pathways. (From Melnikova: Nat Rev Drug Discov 8:353, 2009.)

heparin is basically fragments of unfractionated heparin, but has less inhibitory activity against thrombin than unfractionated heparin.

How is this effect best quantified and monitored? One of the most common coagulation tests is prothrombin time, which assesses the intrinsic clotting pathway, consisting of tissue factor and factor VII, and the common pathway, consisting of factors II, V, X, and fibrinogen. Another coagulation test, the activated partial thromboplastin time, or aPTT, assesses the integrity of the extrinsic coagulation pathway, which consists of prekallikrein, factors XII, XI, IX, and VIII, and the final pathway. Another test that is often used is the activated whole blood clotting test (ACT), which is much faster than aPTT and can be performed at the bedside, in the operating room, or neuroradiology suite. The ACT is less sensitive to low-molecular-weight heparin but can also be used to monitor treatment with dalteparin.

Maintenance IV heparin therapy should result in 1.5–2.5 times control value of the aPTT, and doses are often continuously adjusted using hospital practice nomograms. Patients with a deficiency of antithrombin III are resistant to heparin and require increasing doses.[4]

REVERSAL OF ANTICOAGULATION

The practice of discontinuation of anticoagulation is variable, and major issues quickly surface. Discontinuation of anticoagulation in some patients with cerebral hemorrhage (traumatic or nontraumatic) may expose them to risks. The risk associated with discontinuation of anticoagulation depends on whether a mechanical heart valve, in particular mitral valve, is present.[3,51] As early as day one, the patient is at risk of valve thrombosis that may be rapidly life threatening. Echocardiography is helpful to monitor mitral valve function, and transthoracic echocardiography is often good enough because the mitral valve is close to the surface. Sudden stoppage of leaflet movement indicates thrombus that requires immediate resumption with IV heparin (may be very successful in resolving the thrombus in 1–2 days) or surgical replacement (less attractive option).

Aside from patients with a metallic valve, the risk of thromboembolism is usually assessed using the so-called CHADS2 score, which is made up of congestive heart failure (1 point), hypertension (1 point), age >75 years (1 point), diabetes mellitus (1 point), and prior stroke (2 points). A CHADS2 score of 5–6 has a high risk of arterial or venous thromboembolism when anticoagulation is discontinued. The risk is low with a CHADS2 score of 0–2.

Also increasing the risk of thromboembolism after discontinuation of warfarin is a recent (within three months) history of venous thromboembolism the presence of active cancer or recurrent venous thromboembolism. If a venous thromboembolism has occurred more than a year ago and there are no other risk factors, it does not seem to be concerning when anticoagulation is suddenly discontinued.

Empirically, it appears that discontinuation of warfarin for 7 days may be quite safe in most patients. After this interval resumption of anticoagulation also does not appreciably increase the risk of rehemorrhage.

There are many drugs that can be used to reverse warfarin, and they all have their important characteristics.[45] Table 8.1 summarizes the characteristics of these drugs in detail, including vitamin K, fresh frozen plasma, prothrombin complex concentrate, and recombinant factor VIIa.

Vitamin K enhances the production in the liver of factors II, VII, IX, and X; however, it takes up to 4–6 hours to produce an effect, with a maximal effect after 36 hours. Vitamin K is far less effective in patients with severe hepatic failure because these patients are not able to mount a response. Vitamin K is administered preferably intravenously because subcutaneous vitamin K has an erratic response. Vitamin K is usually administered in an intravenous dose of 10 mg and because of its effect, physicians should appreciate that anticoagulation may be difficult to regulate for up to 2 weeks. Vitamin K continues to be used in combination with fresh frozen plasma, but vitamin K is not necessary when using prothrombin complex concentrate or recombinant factor VIIa.

Table 8.1 **Therapeutic Options for Reversal of Vitamin K Antagonist Therapy**

Options	Vitamin K	Fresh Frozen Plasma	Prothrombin Complex Concentrate	Recombinant Factor VIIa
Rationale	Promotes syntheses of factors II, VII, IX, and X	Replaces factor II, VII, IX, and X. Contains fibrinogen, von Willebrand factor, antithrombin	Contains factor II, VII, IX, X, and proteins S and C	Contains factor VIIa
Dose	5–10 mg IV	10–30 mL/kg, IV Optimal dose is unknown	8–30 IE/kg IV dependent on body weight, initial and target INR	20–30 mcg/kg IV
Time to effect	4–6 h	variable	30 min	30 min
Duration/ Half life	Effect on reversal last until INR is within therapeutic interval again	T ½: 1.5–2 days	T ½: 6–8 h	T ½: <60 min

INR, international normalized ratio. *Source:* From reference 45.

Fresh frozen plasma includes factors II, VII, IX, and X and also has antithrombin III, fibrinogen, and von Willebrand factor. Usually a volume of 10–30 mL/kg is administered. The thawing of fresh frozen plasma may take 30–45 minutes. Fresh frozen plasma is also blood-group specific, although ABRhD fresh frozen plasma is often used, obviating any need for blood typing.[21]

Fresh frozen plasma has many drawbacks. One concern is the long delay until INR normalizes, with a mean time interval between admission and INR normalization of 12 hours (Figure 8.2). With fresh frozen plasma, there is a risk of rebound increase in INR due to faster decay of used coagulation factors in fresh frozen plasma.

Most concerning is that fresh frozen plasma may damage the heart and lungs. There is a risk of transfusion-associated cardiac overload syndrome (TACO) or transfusion-related acute lung injury (TRALI).[7] TACO usually is related to the rate of infusion and the total volume of blood product that has been transfused. Typically patients develop dyspnea, hypertension, and tachypnea and, on auscultation, have significant crackles and rales. If brain natriuretic peptide is measured, it is increased. A chest X-ray often shows development of pulmonary edema and also other features of congestive heart failure. TACO occurs on average in patients who have received four or more units of fresh frozen plasma and when the rate was approximately 500 mL/h before the reaction occurred.[35] There is a quick and effective response to aggressive diuresis and it may require short-term furosemide infusion.

TRALI can occasionally occur, with some series claiming one in four patients.[7] This condition is dramatic, with a sudden severe hypoxemia and pulmonary edema. TRALI characteristically occurs within six hours of transfusion but may be seen earlier if prior transfusions have been administered. Most patients survive TRALI with supportive measures (mechanical ventilation with high positive end-expiratory pressure, but mortality from cardiovascular collapse has occured.

Recombinant factor VIIa is more commonly used in emergency departments but may soon be replaced by prothrombin complex. Recombinant factor VIIa binds

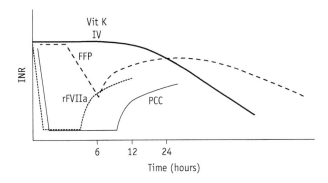

Figure 8.2 Elimination of drugs that reverse anticoagulation.

to the platelet surface and promotes factor X activation and thrombin generation, but only where platelets are localized at the site of injury (the "a" in factor
VII stands for activation of the coagulation process). Despite correction of INR,
recombinant factor VIIa corrects the warfarin-induced decrease in factor VII
activity, but not other factors. The downside of recombinant factor VIIa are that
it does not reverse other factors, may carry a risk of thromboembolic adverse
effects, and has a short half-life of less than an hour. Nonetheless, recombinant
factor VIIa is able to reverse INR within 10 minutes.[42]

Prothrombin complex contains not only vitamin K–dependent clotting factors II, VII, IX, and X but also coagulation inhibitors proteins C and S. Many
studies have found that a simple combined reversal using IV vitamin K and
30–50 units/kg of prothrombin complex concentrates (PCC) will correct the
INR rapidly.[16,31]

In general, looking at the effect on INR, a solution of 60 mL of PCC is similar to 1,500 mL of fresh frozen plasma. Significant fluid overload thus can be
prevented using PCC. The dose of PCC is dependent on the INR but is usually
started at 25–30 IU/kg IV with a maximal rate of infusion of 3 mL/min. This is
adequate in most patients presenting with anticoagulation associated hemorrhages, but up to 60 IU/kg may be needed in extreme INRs (INR >10). To correct
an abnormal INR, many hospital protocols have linked 0.5 increase of INR with
5 IU/kg of PCC (in other words, INR 2.0–2.5 give 30 IU/kg; INR 2.5–3.0 give 35
IU/kg, etc.). Just choosing a high dose (>50 IU/kg) not only may be costly but
also can unnecessarily increase thromboembolic complications. PCC is associated with venous and arterial thromboembolic events that usually include deep
venous thrombosis, but cerebral infarction and bilateral renal infarction have
also been reported.

PCC has become the treatment of choice for emergency reversal of vitamin
K anticoagulants, but a better analysis of thromboembolic risk is necessary.[38]
Rapid correction with PCC is expected in virtually all patients, but there is
no evidence that rapid reversal impacts cerebral hematoma growth, let alone
outcome.[14]

One other circumstance needs to be discussed. Direct thrombin inhibitors
are the newer oral anticoagulation drugs. Dabigatran is currently approved
in the United States, and the oral factor Xa inhibitor rivaroxaban is approved
for venous thromboembolism after orthopedic surgery and for stroke prevention and atrial fibrillation. Apixaban is an oral Xa inhibitor and is approved
in Europe for venous thromboembolism and will likely be approved for atrial
fibrillation in the United States. These anticoagulants inhibit thrombin factor
(factor IIa or factor Xa). The problem with these new anticoagulants is that
none of the currently used methods to reverse anticoagulation could possibly have an effect because these drugs inhibit a single clotting factor (IIa or
Xa).[10,11,15,52] Vitamin K administration also has no role. There are significant
concerns with the emergent reversal of these new oral anticoagulants.

In Practice

All this taken together the management is to anticoagulate or to reverse anticoagulation and to assess long term risks. To do so means following a few simple rules.

TO ANTICOAGULATE

Weight-based nomograms have assisted in rapidly anticoagulating the patient[41] (Table 8.2). Usually this consists of an initial bolus of 80 units/kg/h, followed by an infusion of 18 units/kg/h, and then adjustment after aPTT. The first aPTT should be measured 6 hours after administration.[12,24] Measuring too early will lead to falsely elevated aPTT. If high-dose heparin is needed to fully anticoagulate the patient, or if there is an inability to get to a desired aPTT number, other options are available, including the use of argatroban.

Low-molecular-weight heparins (LMWH) have advantages over unfractionated heparin: LMWH have a greater bioavailability, and longer duration of anticoagulation effect (Table 8.3).[36,50] LMWH is also much less likely to cause immune-mediated thrombocytopenia.[6,13,48] LMWH can be tested by antifactor Xa. The target range—measured 4 hours after dosing—is 0.6–1.0 IU/mL with twice-daily use.

IV heparinization is usually safe and easy to titrate. The most concerning complication is heparin-induced thrombocytopenia (HIT). The diagnosis of HIT should only be considered if symptoms occur approximately five days after exposure (earlier if there has been prior use of heparin). Thrombi on

Table 8.2 **Weight-Based Heparin Nomogram**

Start:	Bolus of heparin, 80 units/kg IV		
	Heparin infusion, 18 units/kg/h (20,000 units in 500 mL of D5W is 40 units/mL)		
Measure:	aPTT 6 hours after bolus		
Adjust:	aPTT, seconds	Bolus, U/kg	New infusion rate, U/kg/hour
	<35	80	22
	35–45	40	20
	46–70	No	18
	71–90	No	16
	>90	No	*15* (stop after 1 hour)

Administration of warfarin, 5–10 mg, can be started on the second day of heparin therapy with long-term anticoagulation. Complete blood count with platelet count is done every 3 days to detect HIT. D5W, 5% dextrose in water; aPTT, activated partial thromboplastin time. *Source:* Modified from reference 41.

Table 8.3 **Pros and Cons of UFH and/LMWH**

LMWH	• Expensive
	• Protamine reversal not fully achieved
	• Not used in renal failure
UFH	• Protamine works rapidly (1 mg for each 100 units of heparin)
	• Much shorter half life than LMWH

LMWH: Low molecular weight heparin; UFH: unfractionated heparin.
Source: From references 36 and 50.

central catheters may be the first noticed sign, and most thrombi remain venous. Thrombocytopenia is usually in the 20,000–100,000 range. Anti-PR4 antibodies can be measured, and either lepirudin or fondaparinux can be used as an alternative for heparin.

If long-term anticoagulation is necessary, warfarin is initiated once heparin is started. Warfarin should ideally be overlapped with heparin for a minimum of five days until INR is within the therapeutic range, usually between 2 and 3.[25,26] Anticoagulation with IV heparin can be maintained for weeks; in many patients, however, transitioning to oral warfarin is initiated early. The main reason for postponing warfarin is anticipated invasive tests or surgical procedures that would require reversal. Warfarin is usually started with 2 days and with 5–10 mg followed by INR measurement and further adjustment to doses that vary from 1 to 10 mg daily.[49] Causes of excessive overanticoagulation are heart failure, diarrhea, fever, and impaired liver function.[37] Falsely elevated INRs can be explained by heparin in the blood sample and when blood is taken from an indwelling central venous catheter contaminated with heparin.

TO REVERSE ANTICOAGULATION

American Heart Association and Neurocritical Care Society recommendations have published recommendations in cerebral hematoma.[2,33] Reversal of warfarin is typically initiated in a patient with INR ≥1.5.[32] Reversal may involve the use of fresh frozen plasma and intravenous vitamin K (10 mg, typically), but recombinant factor VIIa or prothrombin complex concentrate is preferred.[18,22,29,42,45] Current guidelines recommend, next to vitamin K 10 mg intravenously, infusion of 4-factor PCC in combination with fresh frozen plasma or recombinant human factor VIIa. The exact dose of factor VIIa is not known, but most studies have shown that factor VIIa dosed at 10–50 mcg/kg was effective in reversing anticoagulation-associated intracranial hemorrhage. It should be noted that the half-life of factor VIIa is approximately two hours. Infusion of a high dose of factor VIIa—starting at 80 mcg/kg in patients with spontaneous intracranial hemorrhage—significantly increases the risk of arterial and venous thrombosis. This increase is not apparent with infusion of a dose of 20 mcg/kg or less.[19,22,23]

Benefits of PCCs include a short amount of time to normalize INR (usually <30 minutes), little volume of infusion, and administration of all vitamin K–dependent coagulation factors.[44] Another compelling argument to use PCC is that it lasts longer than recombinant factor VIIa and less additional fresh frozen plasma might be needed.

Whether platelet transfusions are needed in patients with cerebral hemorrhage and prior antiplatelet use is unresolved, but one study suggested improvement on platelet activity assay with two packs (containing 6 units and also known as a 6-pack) of apheresis platelets.[34,47] Transfusion of 6 units of platelets should raise the platelet count by 60,000/uL—1 unit increases by 10,000 uL. A considerable number of donor units may be needed to reverse the combined antiaggregant effect of aspirin and clopidogrel. One study in volunteers found 10 donor units for 300 mg, but only 15 donor units for 600 mg of clopidogrel were needed to completely reverse the platelet effects, thus suggesting a nonlinear therapeutic effect.[46]

Reversal of thrombin inhibitors has not been clearly established.[30] Recent guidance has been published that suggests a combination of supportive care, discontinuation of the drug, and possible PCC or hemodialysis. Supportive care would imply blood transfusions in patients who are actively bleeding, maintenance of renal function, identification of the bleeding source, and possible surgical intervention if needed. After the drug is discontinued, the anticoagulant effect is absent after 2 days. Activated charcoal could be is administered, if the drug was taken within hours of presentation. Hemodialysis and hemoperfusion can be considered in patients with impaired renal function that will cause more difficulty with clearing of the drug; however, it is not effective with apixaban or rivaroxaban because they are highly protein bound. Factor VIIa does not reverse the anticoagulant effect, but PCC has been shown to normalize the prothrombin time (PT) in normal volunteers. It is unclear whether it is effective to stop bleeding, but it has been used in emergency situations (Table 8.4).

Restarting anticoagulation is an additional concern and risks are unknown.[8,9] The use of heparin in a patient with prior acute intracranial hemorrhage has been poorly studied, with very few studies available. When low-molecular-weight heparin is started within 96 hours of intracranial hemorrhage onset, no increase in hematoma enlargement has been documented in patients with acute intracranial hemorrhage.[27] Restarting antiplatelets is common (1/3 in one study[37]) after cerebral hemorrhage with no increased risk for recurrent cerebral hematomas.

Table 8.4 **Suggestions for Reversal of New Oral Anticoagulants**

	Apixaban	Dabigatran	Rivaroxaban
Oral activated charcoal	Yes	Yes	Yes
Hemodialysis	No	Yes	No
Hemoperfusion with activated charcoal	Possible	Yes	Possible
Fresh frozen plasma	No	No	No
Factor VIIa	Unclear	Unclear	Unclear
3-factor PCC	Unclear	Unclear	Unclear
4-factor PCC	Possible	Possible	Possible

Source: Adapted from reference 28.

By the Way

Causes of Unstable INR
- Drug malabsorption (tube feeding, ileus)
- Transfusion may lower INR
- Hemodialysis—removal of high protein binding drugs (albumin)
- Plasmapheresis—altering of high-protein-binding drugs
- Prior high IV-dose of vitamin K (>10 mg)
- Drug interaction
- Wrong dose, missed dose, or extra dose

Anticoagulation Strategies by the Numbers

- 90% of patients treated with PCC will have INR corrected within an hour
- 20% of patients may develop a transfusion-associated cardiac overload
- 10% of patients treated with fresh frozen plasma and vitamin K have INR corrected within 3–6 hours
- 1% of patients treated with PCC have a thrombolic event
- <1% of patients may develop a transfusion-related acute lung injury

Putting It All Together

- Warfarin remains the main anticoagulant to use, dabigatran may become an alternative.
- Heparin is mostly used for prophylaxis or when thromboembolic complications have occurred.
- Fresh frozen plasma and vitamin K is not the first line of treatment in patients with cerebral hemorrhage prone to deterioration.
- Reversal of warfarin preferably is done with PCC or factor VIIa in a patient with a high INR.
- Acute reversal of direct thrombin inhibitors is not possible.

References

1. Adams HP Jr, del Zoppo G, Alberts MJ, et al. Guidelines for the early management of adults with ischemic stroke: a guideline from the American Heart Association/American Stroke Association Stroke Council, Clinical Cardiology Council, Cardiovascular Radiology and Intervention Council, and the Atherosclerotic Peripheral Vascular Disease and Quality of Care Outcomes in Research Interdisciplinary Working Groups. *Stroke* 2007;38:1655–1711.
2. Andrews CM, Jauch EC, Hemphill JC 3rd, et al. Emergency neurological life support: intracerebral hemorrhage. *Neurocrit Care* 2012;17: S37–S46.
3. Amin AG, Ng J, Hsu W, et al. Postoperative anticoagulation in patients with mechanical heart valves following surgical treatment of subdural hematomas. *Neurocrit Care* 2013;19:90–94.
4. Baglin T, Barrowcliffe TW, Cohen A, et al. Guidelines on the use and monitoring of heparin. *Br J Haematol* 2006;133:19–34.
5. Baglin T. Management of warfarin (coumarin) overdose. *Blood Rev* 1998;12:91–98.
6. Becker PS, Miller VT. Heparin-induced thrombocytopenia. *Stroke* 1989;20:1449–1459.
7. Benson AB, Moss M, Silliman CC. Transfusion-related acute lung injury (TRALI): a clinical review with emphasis on the critically ill. *Br J Haematol* 2009;147:431–443.
8. Butler AC, Tait RC. Restarting anticoagulation in prosthetic heart valve patients after intracranial hemorrhage: a 2-year follow-up. *Br J Haematol* 1998;103:1064–1066.
9. Claassen DO, Kazemi N, Zubkov AY, et al. Restarting anticoagulation therapy after warfarin-associated intracerebral hemorrhage. *Arch Neurol* 2008;65:1313–1318.
10. Cotton BA, McCarthy JJ, Holcomb JB. Acutely injured patients on dabigatran. *N Engl J Med* 2011;365:2039–2040.
11. Crowther MA, Warkentin TE. Managing bleeding in anticoagulated patients with a focus on novel therapeutic agents. *J Thromb Haemost* 2009;7:107–110.
12. Cruickshank MK, Levine MN, Hirsh J, et al. A standard heparin nomogram for the management of heparin therapy. *Arch Intern Med* 1991;151:333–337.
13. Cuker A. Recent advances in heparin-induced thrombocytopenia. *Curr Opin Hematol* 2011;18:315–322.
14. Dowlatshahi D, Butcher KS, Asdaghi N, et al. Poor prognosis in warfarin-associated intracranial hemorrhage despite anticoagulation reversal. *Stroke* 2012;43:1812–1817.
15. Eerenberg ES, Kamphuisen PW, Sijpkens MK, et al. Reversal of rivaroxaban and dabigatran by prothrombin complex concentrate: a randomized, placebo-controlled, crossover study in healthy subjects. *Circulation* 2011;124:1573–1579.

16. Evans G, Luddington R, Baglin T. Beriplex P/N reverses severe warfarin-induced overanti-coagulation immediately and completely in patients presenting with major bleeding. *Br J Haematol* 2001;115:998–1001.

17. Flynn RW, MacDonald TM, Murray GD, et al. Prescribing antiplatelet medicine and subsequent events after intracerebral hemorrhage. *Stroke* 2010;41:2606–2611.

18. Freeman WD, Brott TG, Barrett KM, et al. Recombinant factor VIIa for rapid reversal of warfarin anticoagulation in acute intracranial hemorrhage. *Mayo Clin Proc* 2004;79:1495–500.

19. Gabriel DA, Carr M, Roberts HR. Monitoring coagulation and the clinical effects of recombinant factor VIIa. *Semin Hematol* 2004;41:20–24.

20. Geerts WH, Bergqvist D, Pineo GF, et al. Prevention of venous thromboembolism: American College of Chest Physicians Evidence-Based Clinical Practice Guidelines (8th edition). *Chest* 2008;133:381S–453S.

21. Goldstein JN, Thomas SH, Frontiero V, et al. Timing of fresh frozen plasma administration and rapid correction of coagulopathy in warfarin-related intracerebral hemorrhage. *Stroke* 2006;37:151–155.

22. Goodnough LT, Shander AS. Recombinant factor VIIa: safety and efficacy. *Curr Opin Hematol* 2007;14:504–509.

23. Hedner U. Dosing with recombinant factor VIIa based on current evidence. *Semin Hematol* 2004;41:35–39.

24. Hirsh J, Anand SS, Halperin JL, et al. Guide to anticoagulant therapy: Heparin: a statement for healthcare professionals from the American Heart Association. *Circulation* 2001;103:2994–3018.

25. Hirsh J, Anand SS, Halperin JL, Fuster V; American Heart Association. Guide to anticoagulant therapy: heparin: a statement for healthcare professionals from the American Heart Association. *Circulation* 2001;103:2994–3018.

26. Hirsh J, Dalen J, Anderson DR, et al. Oral anticoagulants: mechanism of action, clinical effectiveness, and optimal therapeutic range. *Chest* 2001;119:8S–21S.

27. Iwuchukwu, IO, Mckinney, J, Rosenberg, M. DVT prophylaxis and risk of bleeding in intracerebral hemorrhage. *Ann Neurol* 2009;66:S57.

28. Kaatz S, Kouides PA, Garcia DA, et al. Guidance on the emergent reversal of oral thrombin and factor Xa inhibitors. *Am J Hematol* 2012;87 Suppl 1:S141–S145.

29. Kalina M, Tinkoff G, Gbadebo A, Veneri P, Fulda G. A protocol for the rapid normalization of INR in trauma patients with intracranial hemorrhage on prescribed warfarin therapy. *Am Surg* 2008;74:858–861.

30. Lauer A, Pfeilschifter W, Schaffer CB, Lo EH, Foerch C. Intracerebral hemorrhage associated with antithrombotic treatment: translational insights from experimental studies. *Lancet Neurol* 2013;12:394–405.

31. Lubetsky A, Hoffman R, Zimlichman R, et al. Efficacy and safety of a prothrombin complex concentrate (Octaplex) for rapid reversal of oral anticoagulation. *Thromb Res* 2004;113:371–378.

32. Makris M, van Veen JJ, Maclean R. Warfarin anticoagulation reversal: management of the asymptomatic and bleeding patient. *J Thromb Thrombolysis* 2010;29:171–181.

33. Morgenstern LB, Hemphill JC 3rd, Anderson C, et al. Guidelines for the management of spontaneous intracerebral hemorrhage: a guideline for healthcare professionals from the American Heart Association/American Stroke Association. *Stroke* 2010;41:2108–2129.

34. Naidech AM, Liebling SM, Rosenberg NF, et al. Early platelet transfusion improves platelet activity and may improve outcomes after intracerebral hemorrhage. *Neurocrit Care* 2012;16:82–87.

35. Narick C, Triulzi DJ, Yazer MH. Transfusion-associated circulatory overload after plasma transfusion. *Transfusion* 2012;52:160–165.

36. Noble S, Peters D, Goa K. Enoxaparin: a reappraisal of its pharmacology and clinical applications in the prevention and treatment of thromboembolic disease. *Drugs* 1995;49:388–410.

37. Penning-van Beest FJ, van Meegen E, Rosendaal FR, Stricker BH. Characteristics of anticoagulant therapy and comorbidity related to overanticoagulation. *Thromb Haemost* 2001;86:569–574.

38. Preston FE, Laidlaw ST, Sampson B, Kitchen S. Rapid reversal of oral anticoagulation with warfarin by a prothrombin complex concentrate (Beriplex): efficacy and safety in 42 patients. *Br J Haematol* 2002;116:619–624.

39. Racine E. Differentiation of the low-molecular-weight heparins. *Pharmacotherapy* 2001;21:62S–70S.

40. Ranucci M, Isgrò G, Cazzaniga A, et al. Different patterns of heparin resistance: therapeutic implications. *Perfusion* 2002;17:199–204.

41. Raschke RA, Reilly BM, Guidry JR, et al. The weight-based heparin dosing nomogram compared with a "standard care" nomogram. A randomized controlled trial. *Ann Intern Med* 1993;119:874–881.

42. Rosovsky RP, Crowther MA. What is the evidence for the off-label use of recombinant factor VIIa (rFVIIa) in the acute reversal of warfarin? ASH evidence-based review 2008. *Hematology Am Soc Hematol Educ Program* 2008:36–38.

43. Sandercock PA, Counsell C, Kamal AK. Anticoagulants for acute ischemic stroke. *Cochrane Database Syst Rev* 2008 Oct 8;(4):CD000024.

44. Sarode R, Milling TJ, Refaai MA, Mangione A, Schneider A, Durn BL, Goldstein JN. Efficacy and safety of a 4-factor prothrombin complex concentrate in patients on vitamin K antagonists presenting with major bleeding: a randomized, plasma-controlled, phase IIIb study. *Circulation* 2013; 128:1234–1243.

45. Vang ML, Hvas AM, Ravn HB. Urgent reversal of vitamin K antagonist therapy. *Acta Anaesthesiol Scand* 2011;55:507–516.

46. Vilahur G, Choi BG, Zafar MU, et al. Normalization of platelet reactivity in clopidogrel-treated subjects. *J Thromb Haemost* 2007;5:85–90.

47. Viswanathan A, Rakich SM, Engel C, et al. Antiplatelet use after intracerebral hemorrhage. *Neurology* 2006;66:206–209.

48. Warkentin TE, Greinacher A. Heparin-induced thrombocytopenia: recognition, treatment, and prevention: the Seventh ACCP Conference on Antithrombotic and Thrombolytic Therapy. *Chest* 2004;126:311S–337S.

49. Wells PS, Le Gal G, Tierney S, Carrier M. Practical application of the 10-mg warfarin initiation nomogram. *Blood Coagul Fibrinolysis* 2009;20:403–408.

50. White RH, Ginsberg JS. Low-molecular-weight heparins: are they all the same? *Br J Haematol* 2003;121:12–20.

51. Wijdicks EFM, Schievink WI, Brown RD, et al. The dilemma of discontinuation of anticoagulation therapy for patients with intracranial hemorrhage and mechanical heart valves. *Neurosurgery* 1998;42:769–773.

52. Zhou W, Zorn M, Nawroth P, et al. Hemostatic therapy in experimental intracerebral hemorrhage associated with rivarozaban. *Stroke* 2013;44:771–778.

9

Antimicrobial Stewardship

Even with precautionary policies, acutely ill neurologic patients are at high risk for infections, and many will eventually receive antibiotics during their hospital stay. Extended hospital stays and exposure to intensive care units increase the chance of patients being exposed to multidrug-resistant organisms and to develop antibiotic resistance.

Experts in infectious disease have recognized the six so-called ESKAPE pathogens: *Enterococcus faecium*, *Staphylococcus aureus*, *Klebsiella pneumoniae*, and the gram negative bacilli, *Acinetobacter baumannii*, *Pseudomonas aeruginosa*, and *Enterobacter* species. Of all these organisms, gram-negative bacilli remain the most challenging microbials to keep in check or even eradicate.

Generally speaking—in acutely ill neurologic patients—most healthcare-associated infections are pneumonia, urinary tract infections, neurosurgical infections, or infections associated with devices. Bloodstream infections are far less common and usually seen in fulminant meningoencephalitis or patients in a protracted comatose state—these infections will be associated with increasing mortality if sepsis syndrome emerges. Bloodstream infection rates may also occur in 4–9 cases per 1,000 line days. Most common organisms associated with bloodstream infections are coagulase-negative *Staphylococcus*, *Enterococcus*, and gram-negative organisms.

Bladder and bowel infections are also on the rise. Catheter-associated urinary tract infection rates are steadily increasing, as are bowel infections due to *Clostridium difficile*. It has been known for years that overuse of antibiotics increases the risk of *Clostridium difficile* infections, and they are frequently found in chronically ill patients with associated comorbidity and thus in patients with neurologic disease.

All of these infections can be diminished by infection control programs.[12,16] This includes aggressive surveillance with screening cultures on admission that would include rectal swab, sputum and tracheal aspirate, wounds, gastrostomy tube site, and urine cultures. Proper isolation may prevent further horizontal transmission.

So naturally, one of the critical components of antimicrobial stewardship is to identify multidrug-resistant organisms and antibiotic resistance.[2,3,35] Antibiotic resistance is emerging, but dependent on antibiotic usage—high in regions where antibiotic use is ubiquitous. There is resistance to β-lactam antibiotics, aminoglycosides, and fluoroquinolones among many others, but the best known are methicillin resistant staphylococcus aureus (MRSA), vancomycin-resistant *Enterococcus* (VRE), and penicillin-resistant *Streptococcus pneumonia*. Other problems are the extended-spectrum β-lactonase-producing Enterobacteriaceae, carbapenem-resistant Enterobacteriaceae, and multidrug-resistant *Pseudomonas aeruginosa*.[1,13,19,29,33] Management is difficult because these strains are resistant to penicillin, ampicillin, aminoglycosides, and vancomycin. The newer antibiotics linezolid and quinupristin-dalfopristin have both been approved for MRSA and VRE.

What infection does a neurohospitalist or neurointensivist encounter most often? What common pathogens are seen, and how are they best eradicated? What are the criteria for antibiotic treatment? What are appropriate empiric antibiotic choices? This chapter addresses these issues and to illustrate antimicrobial management.

Principles

Antimicrobial stewardship can be broadly defined as organizing a formulary restriction, order sets and treatment algorithms, incorporation of clinical guidelines, pharmacodynamic dose optimization, and pharmacy-driven programs.[17,25,34,38,39,40] Surveillance includes review of microbiology data, but also infectious rate evaluation. (Table 9.1) The Centers for Disease Control National Healthcare Safety Network (NHSN) publishes a semiannual report (www.cdc.gov) and includes healthcare-associated infections reported voluntarily by NHSN facilities. Such infection control and prevention has been structured in most hospitals and guarantees ongoing surveillance. Quality of care may be measured in appropriateness of antibiotic selection and its use. In the United States it has come so far that guidelines by the Centers for Medicare and Medicaid Services may be used to assess hospital reimbursement.[1,2,11,15]

PATHOGENS AND ANTIBIOTICS

One of the most important core principles is to decide which patient to treat and to treat each patient with the appropriate antimicrobial.[18] Hospitals are known to have quite a high rate of colonization. Obviously one should prevent antimicrobial overuse, misuse, and abuse, but practice in the real world does not seem to work that way, and there is a perception that some practices are seriously concerning.

Table 9.1 **Hospital Metrics to Define Infection Rates**

$$\text{BSI rate} = \frac{\text{Number of BSIs}}{\text{Number of central line days}} \times 1{,}000$$

$$\text{Central line utilization ratio} = \frac{\text{Number of central line days}}{\text{Number of patient days}}$$

$$\text{VAP rate} = \frac{\text{Number of VAPs}}{\text{Number of ventilator days}} \times 1{,}000$$

$$\text{Ventilator utilization ratio} = \frac{\text{Number of ventilator days}}{\text{Number of patient days}}$$

$$\text{CAUTI rate} = \frac{\text{Number of catheter associated UTIs}}{\text{Number of urinary catheter days}} \times 1{,}000$$

$$\text{Urinary catheter utilization ratio} = \frac{\text{Number of urinary catheter days}}{\text{Number of patient days}}$$

$$\% \text{ Prevalence on admission} = \frac{\text{Number of cases for specific MDRO}}{\text{Number of admissions}} \times 100\%$$

$$\% \text{ Point prevalence} = \frac{\text{Number of cases for specific MDRO}}{\text{Patient census for specific day}} \times 100\%$$

$$\text{MDRO transmission rate} = \frac{\text{New positive cultures of specific MDRO}}{\text{Patient days}} \times 1{,}000$$

Multidrug-resistant organism (MDRO.) BSI = bloodstream infection. VAP = ventilator-associated pneumonia. CAUTI = catheter-associated urinary tract infection. *Source:* From reference 7.

Infectious disease specialists have identified the so-called 4 Ds of antimicrobial therapy: the right Drug, right Dose, right Deescalation to pathogen-directed therapy, and right Duration of therapy.[20]

The most common misjudgment is the continuous use of antibiotics in a broad-spectrum pattern without adjusting to culture data. Broad-spectrum antimicrobials may increase gram-negative resistance to carbapenems and cephalosporins, and any patient with antimicrobial resistance has a higher risk of mortality if not substantial additional cost to the patient due to prolonged hospital care.[26,27]

Another core principle is antibiotic prophylaxis—a double-edged sword. Patients who have no infection may never develop infection, but prophylaxis could be needed to prevent an otherwise devastating infection if it were to blossom. Specific indications have been proposed and such prophylaxis may involve not only patients but also family members. (The most well known is prophylaxis for contact of patient admitted with meningococcal meningitis.)[6,14]

Perioperative antimicrobial surgical prophylaxis is only recommended for procedures that have a high rate of postoperative wound infection and are "dirty."

Contaminated craniectomies are expected in patients with severe head injuries (closed or penetrating) and in patients with a major skin excoriation. These neurosurgical procedures are at risk—as are other surgical procedures—of *Staphylococcus* or coagulase-negative *Staphylococcus* infection. This includes any type of craniotomy, spine surgery, or cerebrospinal fluid (CSF) shunting. These patients are best given a single dose of cephalosporin (1–2 g IV) or vancomycin (20 mg/kg) before surgery. (Vancomycin is usually administered in patients previously colonized with MRSA or those allergic to penicillin or cephalosporin.) A craniotomy in itself is not a "dirty" procedure, but unfortunately some practices continue to prescribe broad-spectrum antibiotics after such a procedure. There is generally also no need for prophylactic antibiotics in patients who are undergoing endovascular procedures or stent placement.

Patients with a ventriculostomy are at risk for ventriculitis, a potentially very serious infection. The most frequently isolated bacterial agents in ventriculitis are coagulase negative *Staphylococcus* or *Propionibacterium acnes*.[37] Impregnating the ventricular catheter with rifampin and clindamycin has been suggested to prevent such infection. A recent comparison found no major differences in silver versus antibiotic coating in the rates of infection.[41] Most neurosurgeons agree that subcutaneous tunneling and prophylactic administration of antibiotics may reduce the risk and even prevent infections. Therefore the use of prophylactic antibiotics is not established in patients with a ventriculostomy, but many neurosurgeons prefer prophylactic antibiotics (cefazolin or, when allergic to cefazolin, vancomycin) while the drain is present and perform CSF culture every 3 days or if signs of infection emerge such as fever and a positive Gram stain. (CSF cell count may be an unreliable marker with a device in situ and cultures are needed to make the diagnosis.)

CHOOSING ANTIBIOTICS

The most common pathogens are shown in Table 9.2 for easy reference. The general susceptibility of bacteria to commonly prescribed antibiotics is known and is summarized in Figure 9.1. There are guidelines that can be used in determining the appropriate antibiotic, and some common but essential knowledge is surveyed here primarily to provide a quick update. Treatment of an infectious disease with antibiotics should, however, depend on more specifics and in particular on the susceptibility of the organism to antimicrobials. Tests of antibiotic susceptibility usually report minimum inhibitory concentration semiquantitatively as sensitive, intermediate, or resistant.

Penicillins in general have a spectrum of activity toward gram-positive and gram-negative cocci. (Gram-positive cocci are *Enterococcus*, β-*Streptococcus* [groups A, B, C, and G], *S. pneumoniae*, and *Streptococcus bovis*.) Gram-negative cocci are *Neisseria meningitidis*. Although rarely relevant in the context of acutely ill neurologic patients, penicillins act against gram-positive and gram-negative

Table 9.2 **Common Pathogens**

	Gram Negative	Gram Positive
Rod	Pseudomonas	Nocardia
	Haemophilus	Actinomyces
	Bacteroides	Clostridium
	Fusobacterium	Listeria
	Campylobacter	Lactobacillus
Coccus	Neisseria	Staphylococcus
	Branhamella	Streptococcus

bacilli. The gram-positive bacilli are *Bacillus anthracis, Clostridium perfringens,* and *Clostridium tetani*. Penicillin is also a drug of choice for gram-negative bacilli such as *Pasteurella multocida, Fusobacterium* species, and *Streptobacillus moniliformis*. There are many penicillinase-resistant penicillins; these agents are oxacillin, nafcillin, and dicloxacillin. Its spectrum of activity is for methicillin-sensitive *S. aureus* (MSSA). It is active against most *Streptococci* but has no gram-negative or anaerobic activity.

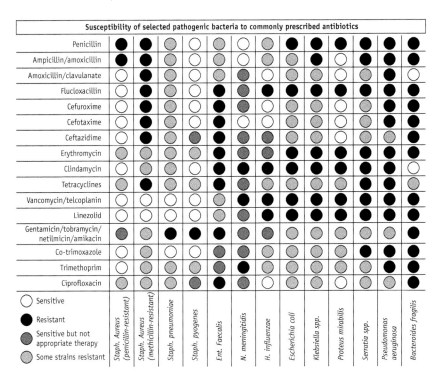

Figure 9.1 Susceptibility of major microorganisms to antibiotics. (Adapted from Warrell D, Cox TM, Firth J, Torok ME. *Textbook of Medicine: Infection*. New York, Oxford University Press, 2012.)

The β-lactam and β-lactamase inhibitor combinations are commonly used. They have a good anaerobic activity and increased activity against β-lactamase-producing organisms such as MSSA. They are not active against MRSA or penicillin-resistant *S. pneumoniae*.

Cephalosporins consist of the first-generation cefazolin, second-generation cefuroxime, and third-generation cefotaxime and ceftriaxone. Fourth-generation cephalosporin cefepime is very active against *P. aeruginosa*, has an improved gram-positive activity toward *S. aureus* and *Pneumococci*, is less likely to induce β-lactamase of *Enterobacter* species, and has very good central nervous system penetration. Its long half-life allows for every-12-hour dosing.

The fluoroquinolones include ciprofloxacin and levofloxacin. These drugs have an excellent tissue penetration with high enteric absorption. It is most active against aerobic gram-negative bacteria, including the Enterobacteriaceae, and active against *Pseudomonas aeruginosa*. It is not reliable for treatment of *Streptococci* such as *S. pneumoniae* infections. Ciprofloxacin is not recommended for initial coverage against respiratory tract infections.

The carbapenems (imipenem and meropenem) have the broadest antibacterial activity of any antibiotic class and have excellent activity against MSSA, *Streptococcus*, and *Enterococcus* species. The carbapenems are very effective but not preferred, and are possibly contraindicated in patients with acute brain injury at risk of seizures, since these antibiotics lower the seizure threshold. The imipenem seizure rates are much higher (3%–33%) than meropenem rates, which are less than 1%, and even the newer carbapenems such as ertapenem may have low risk of seizures.[32]

Vancomycin is the drug of choice for multidrug-resistant gram-positive organisms. Vancomycin has significant toxicity that includes infusion-related pruritus, erythematous rash involving face, neck, and upper body producing a "red man" syndrome. Reducing the rate of infusion and administration of antihistamines before vancomycin infusion can reduce this response. Vancomycin toxicity causing nephrotoxicity is rare but only occurs when used in a high dose (Chapter 10). It is associated with a reversible neutropenia in 2% of the cases.

Linezolid has excellent tissue distribution but has significant adverse effects that include thrombocytopenia and anemia. It is primarily used to treat MRSA and VRE. Tigecycline is a new agent derived from minocycline and is active against many gram-positive, gram-negative, aerobic, and atypical species. It is important to note that it is inactive against *Pseudomonas aeruginosa*.

Finally, fungal infections are best treated with amphotericin B or fluconazole. Amphotericin B has a broad range of activity against yeast and filamentous fungi but has significant nephrotoxicity and can lead to hypoglycemia and hypomagnesemia. Infusion-related fever and phlebitis are unfortunately common. Fluconazole has a very broad spectrum of activity against *Candida* and *Coccidioides* and is commonly used for prophylaxis of candida infections in bone marrow patients or maintenance therapy of cryptococcal meningitis. Another commonly used antifungal is voriconazole, which is active against *Aspergillus*, *Candida*, and *Cryptococcus*, among others, but is not active against mucormycosis.

In Practice

Antimicrobial stewardship leads to uniformity of prescribing guidelines and formularies. However, this may be paradoxically harmful, because resistance occurs if there is no diversity or individualization of prescribing. Similar to the CDC "Get Smart" campaign it is useful to have some important rules (Table 9.3). Unfortunately, use of monotherapy has virtually disappeared, and policies to "cover every possible severe infection" are commonplace. Combination therapies, which usually are initiated to broaden the spectrum, may increase antibiotic resistance. On several occasions, prescribing is inappropriate (the "just in case" argument) or is based on misdiagnosis and poor assessment of the true likelihood of a certain infection.[13,14]

Mundane issues such as regular changing of a white coat or removal of wristwatches reduce contamination with MSSA and MRSA.[4,28] Effective hand hygiene using antibacterial hand rubs has become commonplace and is very effective in killing a range of microorganisms. There is evidence that hand washing may cause cracked skin and dermatitis and increase the risk of colonization with hospital flora, but certain infections require soap and water to provide better hygiene. Still, many infectious disease experts feel that there might be an obsession with hand hygiene and that other measures are far more important. They include antimicrobial prescribing, surveillance, audit and feedback, patient screening and catheter care, isolation when appropriate, reducing occupancy rates, and targeted cleaning.[5,9,30] It has been said that providing sufficiently clean linens for patients every day already improves infection control in a significant manner. Selective digestive and oropharyngeal decontamination continuous to be controversial and its effect of antimicrobial resistance reduction is not completely certain with little endorsement of major societies.[10]

Prevention of intravascular catheter infections include: avoidance of replacing peripheral catheters more frequently than every 72-96 hours, avoidance of removing catheter on the basis of fever only, but most importantly weigh the

Table 9.3 **Core Principles of Antimicrobial Stewardship**

Critically identify need for antibiotic therapy-most do not need
Avoid overlapping therapy—not more effective
Adjust dose and use trough levels for vancomycin—toxicity may quickly occur
Use stop dates—prolonged use is common
Stop antibiotics if no source—often negative blood or sputum cultures
Reconsider perioperative prophylaxis—very few patients need it

risk and benefits of placing them in the first place and avoid the femoral vein for central access.[31]

Physical isolation of patients in a single room has been used, particularly in patients with high-risk microorganisms such as MRSA.[8] It has been considered effective, but the published data is weak and unable to document that the rate of MRSA acquisition can be reduced by isolation of patients. This practice undoubtedly will not change despite unproven benefits.[24,36] Much less appreciated is that avoidance of intubation and even use of noninvasive ventilation reduces the risk of nosocomial pulmonary infections.

Despite the culture of overprescribing, there has been a concern about delay in initiating antibiotic treatment; some studies have found that a delay exceeding 36 hours increases the risk of death 100-fold in patients who are suspected of sepsis. However, other studies found that illness severity and immunosuppression are independent predictors; and variables associated with antibiotic policy do not seem to be associated with mortality. This does not negate the fact that antibiotics should be prescribed immediately and could be quite effective, but whether it impacts on outcome remains unproven.

The time period that antibiotics are used can also be scrutinized. Most of the antibiotic courses are simply empirical, lasting 7 to 14 days. Stopping rules are useful and often include careful assessment of clinical effect. Short-term courses appear to be as effective, with good clinical response. To illustrate that, one important study found that 8 days of antibiotics for ventilator-associated pneumonia was just as effective as 15 days of treatment, with more resistant organisms emerging in the 15-day-treatment patient group.[7]

TREATMENT OF INFECTIONS

The approach to antibiotic therapy is usually four-fold: it should define the host, define the syndrome, define the potential microbiology, and define antimicrobial therapy. Pulmonary infections predominate in acutely ill neurologic patients and therefore need a more detailed discussion.

Empiric treatment of a hospitalized patient with a healthcare-acquired pneumonia and low-risk factors for multidrug-resistant organisms is therefore typically levofloxacin or moxifloxacin, or a combination of a select β-lactam (ceftriaxone, cefotaxime, ertapenem, or ampicillin) plus a select macrolide (azithromycin). An empiric regimen for hospitalized patients with healthcare-acquired pneumonia and risk factors for multidrug-resistant organisms includes several options such as antipseudomonal cephalosporin (cefepime) or antipseudomonal carbapenem, or piperacillin and tazobactam and antipseudomonal fluoroquinolones, or aminoglycoside with vancomycin or linezolid. In patients who have been admitted to an intensive care unit, a combination therapy is often used, with a select β-lactam (ceftriaxone, cefotaxime, or ampicillin/sulbactam) plus fluoroquinolone (levofloxacin or moxifloxacin). An antipseudomonal β-lactam is ciprofloxacin combined with an aminoglycoside (Table 9.4). If there is a concern that the pneumonia is community acquired through MRSA, vancomycin or linezolid should be added to the regimen.

The options for treatment of *P. aeruginosa* include cephalosporins (e.g., cefepime, ceftazidime), fluoroquinolones (e.g., ciprofloxacin, meropenem, and

Table 9.4 **Recommendations for Community-Acquired Pneumonia**

Non-ICU patients	ICU Patients	Non-ICU Patients with Pseudomonal Risk[a]
β-lactam (IV or IM)[b] + macrolide (IV or oral)[c]	Macrolide (IV)[f] + either β-lactam (IV)[g] or antipneumococcal/ antipseudomonal β-lactam (IV)[h]	Antipneumococcal/ antipseudomonal β-lactam (IV)[h] + antipseudomonal quinolone (IV or oral)[j]
Antipneumococcal quinolone monotherapy (IV or oral)[d]	Antipneumococcal quinolone (IV)[I] or antipseudomonal quinolone (IV)[j] + either β-lactam (IV)[g] or antipneumococcal/ antipseudomonal β-lactam (IV)[h]	Antipseudomonal β-lactam (IV)[h] + aminoglycoside (IV)[k] + either antipneumococcal quinolone (IV or oral)[d] or macrolide (IV or oral)[c]
β-Lactam (IV or IM)[b] + doxycycline (IV or oral) or tigecyline monotherapy (IV) or macrolide monotherapy (IV or oral)[c,e]	Antipneumococcal/ antipseudomonal β-lactam (IV)[h] + aminoglycoside (IV)[k] + either antipneumococcal quinolone (IV)[j] or macrolide (IV)[f]	Aztreonam (IV or IM)[l] + antipneumococcal quinolone (IV or oral)[d,l] + aminoglycoside (IV)[k,l] aztreonam (IV or IM)[l,m] + levofloxacin 750 mg (IV or oral)[l]

NOTE: ICU, intensive care unit; IM, intramuscular; IV, intravenous.

   a. These antibiotics are acceptable for non-ICU patients with pseudomonal risk only.

   b. Ceftriaxone, cefotaxime, ampicillin/sulbactam, ertapenem.

   c. Erythromycin, clarithromycin, azithromycin.

   d. Levofloxacin 750 mg, moxifloxacin, gemifloxacin.

   e. If <65 years of age with no risk factors for drug-resistant *Pneumococcus*.

   f. Erythromycin, azithromycin.

   g. Ceftriaxone, cefotaxime, ampicillin/sulbactam.

   h. Cefepime, imipenem, meropenem, piperacillin/tazobactam, doripenem.

   i. Levofloxacin 750 mg, moxifloxacin.

   j. Ciprofloxacin, levofloxacin 750 mg.

   k. Gentamicin, tobramycin, amikacin.

   l. If documented β-lactam allergy.

   m. For patients with renal insufficiency

Source: The Joint Commission, 2011. Reprinted with permission.

imipenem), aminoglycosides (e.g., tobramycin and gentamicin), aztreonam, and perhaps most frequently a piperacillin and tazobactam combination.

Aspiration pneumonia is very common in neurology patients. The expected organisms are shown in Table 9.5, although a mixed flora is typical with cultures. Aspiration pneumonia is typically treated with fluoroquinolone (levofloxacin or moxifloxacin) combined with metronidazole. Knowing these preferences, antimicrobials need to be deescalated on the basis of culture results, and typically the duration of therapy is 7 days if the patient responds and the etiologic agent is not *P. aeruginosa*.

Urinary tract infections are very common in neurologic patients. Urinary tract infection is typically diagnosed on the basis of urine culture more than 10,000 cfu/mL in urine and the presence of clumps of bacteria. Common pathogens are *Escherichia coli*, *Klebsiella*, *Enterobacter*, *Pseudomonas mirabilis*, and *Staphylococcus aureus*. Uncomplicated urinary tract infection (pyelonephritis) is treated with ciprofloxacin 400 mg IV q 12 hours, or levofloxacin 500 mg IV q 25 hours, an aminoglycoside and ampicillin, extended-spectrum cephalosporin, or carbapenem, depending on local susceptibilities. If *Enterococcus* is suspected by Gram stain, ampicillin 1–2 g IV q 6 hours or vancomycin with recent penicillin use should be considered.

Also commonly encountered is an intravascular catheter-related infection.[29] The diagnosis is usually based on microbial growth from blood cultures drawn through the catheter hub. A patient is typically treated for 10–14 days, but occasionally up to 4–6 weeks after removal of the infected catheter in certain circumstances. The choice of antibiotics depends on which organism is present. Surveillance studies have found that the use of multiple lines increases the risk, but five simple steps—hand washing, use of full barrier precautions during insertion of central venous catheter, cleansing the skin with chlorhexidine, avoiding the femoral site, and removing unnecessary catheters—have a great effect on the rate of catheter-related bloodstream infections.[34]

Table 9.5 **Commonly Found Organisms in Aspiration Pneumonia**

Aspiration Pneumonia in Acutely Ill Neurologic Patient	
Community acquired	Healthcare acquired
Haemophilus influenzae	Anaerobes *Streptococcus*
Streptococcus pneumonia	Other otopharyngeal
Anaerobes	*Streptococcus aureus*
Other otopharyngeal	*Enterobacteriaceae*
Streptococcus	*Pseudomonas aeruginosa*

TREATMENT OF ANTIBIOTIC-RESISTANT INFECTIONS

These are complex problems and require input from an infectious disease consultant. In general, the most important consideration for treatment of MRSA simply has to do with whether the infection is serious. A serious infection would require a multipronged treatment with vancomycin, linezolid, daptomycin, or tigecycline. A recent suggested approach for the management of patients with infection by multidrug-resistant gram-negative pathogens is summarized in Table 9.6.

VRE is common, and isolates may have up to 80% VRE. Patients with VRE are usually treated with linezolid or tigecycline. These are bacteriostatic drugs

Table 9.6 **Suggested Approach to Manage Patients with Serious Infections Due to Multidrug-Resistant Gram-Negative Pathogens[a]**

Organism	First-Line Therapy	Second-Line Therapy
Empirical therapy[b]		
Monomicrobial infection	Carbapenem Tigecycline (not with urinary tract infections) with or without an antipseudomonal agent	Piperacillin-tazobactam (low inoculum) Colistin
Mixed gram-positive and gram-negative infection	Anti-MRSA agent plus a carbapenem Tigecycline (not with urinary tract infections) with or without an antipseudomonal agent	Anti-MRSA agent plus piperacillin-tazobactam (low inoculum) Anti-MRSA agent plus colistin
Directed therapy[c]		
ESBL-producing Enterobacteriaceae	Carbapenems Piperacillin-tazobactam (low inoculum) Fosfomycin (oral formulation for simple urinary tract infections)	Tigecycline (not in urinary tract infections) Fluoroquinolone Colistin
Carbapenemase-producing Enterobacteriaceae	Tigecycline Colistin	Fosfomycin (parenteral formulation)
Multidrug-resistant *Pseudomonas aeruginosa*	Antipseudomonal agent (among carbapenems, use doripenem or meropenem)	Colistin Combination therapy

a. ESBL = extended-spectrum β-lactamase; MRSA = methicillin-resistant *Staphylococcus aureus*.

b. Local susceptibility patterns should be taken into consideration before deciding on empirical therapy.

c. Based on available culture and susceptibility results.

Source: With permission from reference 22.

against *Enterococci* and *Staphylococci* and have been approved for VRE infections. Linezolid has significant side effects that include bone marrow suppression and serotonin syndrome (Chapter 10).

MRSA is another important infection. These infections are typically treated with vancomycin, daptomycin, or linezolid. Resistant gram-negative organisms are typically seen with *Klebsiella pneumoniae* but also with *Acinetobacter* and *P. aeruginosa*. These infections are complicated and usually treated with prolonged infusions with β-lactams.

The transmission rates of multidrug-resistant organisms are usually in outbreaks that are occasionally reported to the Centers for Disease Control and Prevention. In general, carbapenems are considered the first-line treatment in infections caused by extended-spectrum β-lactamase producing organisms. Usually this involves imipenem at 500 mg IV every 6 hours up to 1 g IV every 8 hours. An alternative drug is tigecycline 100 mg loading dose IV followed by 50 mg IV every 12 hours, which is quite active against Enterobacteriaceae. Another problematic infection is carbapenem-resistant Enterobacteriaceae. The option here again is tigecycline or cholistine.

Multidrug-resistant *P. aeruginosa*, defined as resistance against two or more classes of antibiotics, has emerged and has become problematic in any intensive care setting.[21,22,23] These infections are complex to treat, but the options are antipseudomonal penicillins such as ticarcillin at a dose of 3 g IV every 4 hours.

By the Way

- Cleaning and disinfection may only remove 50% of nosocomial pathogens
- Many pathogenic microorganisms are on common hospital surfaces
- *C. difficile* can survive disinfectants and detergents.
- Patient admitted to a room with a prior admission containing VRA, VRE, or MRSA is much higher at risk to acquire these organisms.

Healthcare Infections by the Numbers

- 30% of all healthcare infections are urinary tract infections
- 30% of bloodstream infections are due to intravascular infections
- 25% of patients on mechanical ventilator develop pneumonia after 30 days
- 20% of all healthcare infections are pneumoniae
- 10% of all healthcare infections are bloodstream

Putting It All Together

- Healthcare-associated infections are device, procedure, and antibiotic use related
- Hospital-acquired pneumonia is a common concern in acutely ill neurologic patients and determines outcome
- There are multiple effective antibiotics with specific spectrum against certain organisms despite growing multiresistance
- Multidrug-resistant organisms are often seen in outbreaks
- Appropriate use of antibiotics remains a difficult decision for many physicians

References

1. American Thoracic Society; Infectious Diseases Society of America. Guidelines for the management of adults with hospital-acquired, ventilator-associated, and healthcare-associated pneumonia. *Am J Respir Crit Care Med* 2005;171:388–416.
2. Anonymous. Invest to beat the bugs. *BMA News* 2008;27.
3. Berntsen CA, McDermott W. Increased transmissibility of staphylococci to patients receiving an antimicrobial drug. *N Engl J Med* 1960;262:637–642.
4. Bhusal Y, Laza S, Lane TW, Schultz K, Hansen C. Bacterial colonization of wristwatches worn by healthcare personnel. *Am J Infect Control* 2009;37:476–477.
5. Brady RR, Wasson A, Stirling I, McAllister C, Damani NN. Is your phone bugged? The incidence of bacteria known to cause nosocomial infection on healthcare workers' mobile phones. *J Hosp Infect* 2006;62:123–125.
6. Bratzler DW, Houck PM. Antimicrobial prophylaxis for surgery: an advisory statement from the National Surgical Infection Prevention Project. *Clin Infect Dis* 2004;38:1706–1715.
7. Chastre J, Wolf M, Fagon J-Y, et al. Comparison of 8 vs 15 days of antibiotic therapy for ventilator-associated pneumonia in adults. *JAMA* 2003;290:2588–2598.
8. Cepeda JA, Whitehouse T, Cooper B, et al. Isolation of patients in single rooms or cohorts to reduce spread of MRSA in intensive-care units: prospective two-centre study. *Lancet* 2005;365:295–304.
9. Dancer SJ. Pants, policies and paranoia. *J Hosp Infect* 2010;74:10–15.
10. Daneman N, Sarwar S, Fowler RA, Cuthberston BH, SuDDICU Canadian Study Group. Effect of selective decontamination on antimicrobial resistance in intensive care units: a systematic review and meta-analysis. *Lancet Infect Dis* 2013;13:328–341.
11. Davey P, Brown E, Fenelon L, et al. Systematic review of antimicrobial drug prescribing in hospitals. *Emerg Infect Dis* 2006;12:211–216.
12. Doron S, Davidson LE. Antimicrobial stewardship. *Mayo Clin Proc* 2011;86:1113–1123.
13. Edgeworth J. Intravascular catheter infections. *J Hosp Infect* 2009;73:323–330.
14. Enzler MJ, Berbari E, Osmon DR. Antimicrobial prophylaxis in adults. *Mayo Clin Proc* 2011;86:686–701.
15. File TM Jr, Solomkin JS, Cosgrove SE. Strategies for improving antimicrobial use and the role of antimicrobial stewardship programs. *Clin Infect Dis* 2011;53 Suppl 1:S15–S22.
16. Galvin S, Dolan A, Cahill O, Daniels S, Humphreys H. Microbial monitoring of the hospital environment: why and how? *J Hosp Infect* 2012;82:143–151.
17. Gould IM. Antibiotic policies to control hospital-acquired infection. *J Antimicrob Chemother* 2008;61:763–765.
18. Gould IM. Antimicrobials: an endangered species? *Int J Antimicrob Agents* 2007;30:383–384.
19. Gould IM. Controversies in infection: infection control or antibiotic stewardship to control healthcare-acquired infection? *J Hosp Infect* 2009;73:386–391.

20. Joseph J, Rodvold KA. The role of carbapenems in the treatment of severe nosocomial respiratory tract infections. *Expert Opin Pharmacother* 2008;9:561–575.

21. Kallen AJ, Srinivasan A. Current epidemiology of multidrug-resistant gram-negative bacilli in the United States. *Infect Control Hosp Epidemiol* 2010;31 Suppl 1:S51–S54.

22. Kallen AJ, Mu Y, Bulens S, et al. Health care-associated invasive MRSA infections, 2005–2008. *JAMA* 2010;304:641–648.

23. Kanj SS, Kanafani ZA. Current concepts in antimicrobial therapy against resistant gram-negative organisms: extended-spectrum beta-lactamase-producing Enterobacteriaceae, carbapenem-resistant Enterobacteriaceae, and multidrug-resistant *Pseudomonas aeruginosa*. *Mayo Clin Proc* 2011;86:250–259.

24. Kirkland KB. Taking off the gloves: toward a less dogmatic approach to the use of contact isolation. *Clin Infect Dis* 2009;48:766–771.

25. Klompas M, Magill S, Robicsek A, et al. Objective surveillance definitions for ventilator-associated pneumonia. *Crit Care Med* 2012;40:3154–3161.

26. Livermore DM. Introduction: the challenge of multiresistance. *Int J Antimicrob Agents* 2007;29:S1–S7.

27. Livermore DM. Minimizing antibiotic resistance. *Lancet Infect Dis* 2005;5:450–459.

28. Loh W, Ng VV, Holton J. Bacterial flora on the white coats of medical students. *J Hosp Infect* 2000;45:65–68.

29. Maki DG, Kluger DM, Crnich CJ. The risk of bloodstream infection in adults with different intravascular devices: a systematic review of 200 published prospective studies. *Mayo Clin Proc* 2006;81:1159–1171.

30. Malnick S, Bardenstein R, Huszar M, Gabbay J, Borkow G. Pajamas and sheets as a potential source of nosocomial pathogens. *J Hosp Infect* 2008;70:89–92.

31. Mermel LA. Prevention of intravascular catheter-related infections. *Ann Intern Med* 2000;132:391–402.

32. Miller AD, Ball A, Bookstaver B, et al. Epileptogenic potential of carbapenem agents: mechanism of action, seizure rates, and clinical considerations. *Pharmacotherapy* 2011;3:408–423.

33. Pronovost P, Needham D, Berenholtz S, et al. An intervention to decrease catheter-related bloodstream infections in the ICU. *N Engl J Med* 2006;355:2725–2732.

34. Prowle JR, Heenen S, Singer M. Infection in the critically ill—questions we should be asking. *J Antimicrob Chemother* 2011;66:ii3–ii10.

35. Sandiumenge A, Diaz E, Rodriguez A, et al. Impact of diversity of antibiotic use on the development of antimicrobial resistance. *J Antimicrob Chemother* 2006;57:1197–1204.

36. Stelfox HT, Bates DW, Redelmeier DA. Safety of patients isolated for infection control. *JAMA* 2003;290:1899–1905.

37. van de Beek D, Drake JM, Tunkel AR. Nosocomial bacterial meningitis. *N Engl J Med* 2010; 362:146–154.

38. Weiss K, Blais R, Fortin A, Lantin S, Gaudet M. Impact of a multipronged education strategy on antibiotic prescribing in Quebec, Canada. *Clin Infect Dis* 2011;53:433–439.

39. Wright MO, Fisher A, John M, Reynolds K, Peterson LR, Robicsek A. The electronic medical record as a tool for infection surveillance: Successful automation of device-days. *Am J Infect Control* 2009;37:364–370.

40. Wright MO. Surveillance: challenges and direction. *Am J Infect Control.* 2012;40:686–687.

41. Winkler KML, Woernie CM, Seule M, et al. Antibiotic-impregnated vs silver-bearing external ventricular catheters: Preliminary results in a randomized controlled trial. *Neurocrit Care* 2013;18:161–165.

10

Troubleshooting: Drug Adverse Effects

Acutely ill neurologic patients may have multiple drug administrations that can lead to interactions and major side effects. This includes drugs specifically for neurologic disorders (i.e., IV immunoglobulin [IVIG], combinations of antiepileptic drugs) or medication that is related to a systemic or infectious complication (i.e., antibiotics). Troubleshooting drug adverse effects—or at least recognizing them and at best avoiding them—is part of providing acute care. The aim of this chapter is to discuss several common categories that should start further measures to prevent ongoing adverse effects. Put less delicately, no physician will be able to grasp the complexity of drug interactions; and fortunately, hospitals have pharmacy databases and competent pharmacists who can easily provide the information sought.

Drug-Induced Effects

Adverse drug effects may be due to drug administration errors, and any hospital environment with a high rate of distractions and interruptions (emergency department and intensive care units) substantially increases the risk. Pharmacists have identified so-called high-alert medications. These drugs (e.g., heparin, neuromuscular blockers, sedatives, and opioids) have a tendency to quickly cause harm if used in an erroneous dose or erroneous infusion rates. Personnel staffing is also a major variable, with increasing complications at night and weekends when staffing may be shortchanged.[20]

Drug-related events remain more common than any other adverse events in the hospital. Clinicians will improve their practice quality if they avoid high-risk drugs, continuously reassess the need for drugs, consider the possibility that a drug may cause laboratory abnormalities or a clinical sign (e.g., fever, swelling), and generally—as part of a daily routine and double check—to be vigilant regarding drug-drug interactions.

DRUG-INDUCED CHANGES IN ELECTROCARDIOGRAM

There has been a renewed interest in drug-associated electrocardiogram (EKG) changes that could potentially be harbingers of a major cardiac arrhythmia.[41] Most concerning is not only that these drugs are noncardiac—eluding recognition by non-cardiologists—but also that most drugs produce subtle QT prolongation, at least initially. Drugs that prolong the QT interval have been associated with increased rates of death in patients in hospital.[23] QT-interval prolongation can be classified as mild (450–470 ms), moderate (470–499 ms), or severe (more than 500 ms).The QT interval is best measured in lead II (in women, QTc interval is 20 ms greater).

QT-interval prolongation is a result of prolonged depolarization, reduced repolarization, or a combination.[29,39] Naturally, any QT prolongation with prior episodes of arrhythmias or prior torsade de pointes (TdP) is a life-threatening disorder.[41] Many cardiac antiarrhythmics can cause QT prolongation; they include amiodarone, sotalol, mexiletine, and propafenone. Cardiac arrhythmias in these drugs can be expected and anticipated, but this is generally not the case with many other drugs. Examples are methadone, haloperidol, and other first-generation antipsychotics and, of greater concern, the second-generation antipsychotics (clozapine, quetiapine, olanzapine, and risperidone) (Table 10.1). Many antimicrobial agents, particularly the macrolides and fluoroquinolones, are notorious for prolongation of QT interval and should be replaced in susceptible patients. Erythromycin has been incidentally linked to TdP.[15, 45]

Another drug-induced EKG change is PR prolongation (or first-degree AV block). The PR interval is increased when it is greater than 0.20 seconds. Besides cardiac drugs such as calcium channel blockers and digoxin, "neurologic drugs" that are well known to cause these changes are lacosamide and cholinesterase

Table 10.1 **Drugs That Can Prolong QT Interval on EKG**

Antiarrhythmic drugs
Calcium channel blockers
Neuroleptics
Tricyclic antidepressants
Lithium
Selective serotonin reuptake inhibitors
Antihistamines
Antibiotics
Tacrolimus
Vasopressors
Adenosine

inhibitors such as neostigmine. PR prolongation may occur with any increased vagal tone. In healthy individuals, it increases the risk of atrial fibrillation and may even lead to pacemaker implantation and, therefore, is not a trivial EKG abnormality. In any of these circumstances, potassium concentration should be carefully monitored. If TdP has been documented, infusing IV magnesium (1–2 grams) is required, with cardiac pacing in recurrent cases.[45]

DRUG-INDUCED ELECTROLYTE ABNORMALITIES

Electrolyte abnormalities are very common in hospitalized patients, and therefore it will be difficult to definitively implicate a drug side effect. Sodium abnormalities—hypo- or hypernatremia—are often a result of osmotic diuretics (mannitol or hypertonic saline), and volume expansion may be followed by volume depletion. Many drugs have been associated with inappropriate antidiuretic hormone (ADH) syndrome such as proton pump inhibitors, cyclophosphamide, morphine, barbiturates, and antidepressants. Hypernatremia is associated with amphotericin B use, but likely through a different mechanism and as a result of nephrogenic diabetes insipidus.

Drug-induced hypokalemia is uncommon and even more difficult to prove owing to potassium's consistent tendency to decline in hospitalized patients.[7] Sympathicomimetics (epinephrine and dobutamine), any diuretic, glucocorticoids, and aminoglycosides may enhance sodium reabsorption at the distal tube and eliminate potassium. Hyperkalemia has been associated with use of β-blockers that inhibit the Na+-K+-ATPase pump, but any of these effects is likely very small. Other electrolyte disorders such as changes in phosphate, calcium, and magnesium may have to do with increased renal secretion. Diuretics and aminoglycosides have each been implicated and thiazides, in particular, may cause marked hypomagnesemia (a full list of drugs has been published).[7]

DRUG-INDUCED NEPHROTOXICITY

The most common cause for iatrogenic nephrotoxicity is the use of intravenous contrast. Contrast may also cause an important allergic response or neurotoxicity. Known contrast allergy is pretreated with prednisone 50 mg p.o. in three doses 12, 6, and 1 hour(s) before administration, combined with diphenhydramine 50 mg p.o. 1 hour before administration. Nephrotoxicity is usually caused by iodinated contrast and theoretically is a preventable complication.[24] Several scoring systems are known. The Mehran scoring system (Table 10.2) uses as parameters the amount of contrast administered, the baseline glomerular filtration rate, hemodynamic instability, congestive heart failure, age, anemia, and diabetes. When the risk category increases, the incidence of contrast-induced nephropathy increases to 70%.

Table 10.2 **Mehran Scoring Based on Risk Factors for Contrast-Induced Nephropathy**

Risk factor	Point value	
Systolic blood pressure <80 mm Hg	5	
Intraarterial balloon pump	5	
Congestive heart failure (class III/IV or history of pulmonary edema)	5	
Age >75 years old	4	
Hematocrit level (<39% for men and <35 % for women	3	
Diabetes	3	
Contrast media volume	1	point for each 100 mL given
Renal insufficiency	4	points for serum creatinine >1.5 g/dL
	2	points for GFR of 40–60 mL/min/1.73 m^2
	4	points for GFR of 20–40 mL/min/1.73 m^2
	6	points for GFR of <20 mL/min/1.73 m^2

Risk score	Risk of CIN	Risk of dialysis
5 or less	7.5%	0.04%
6–10	14.0%	0.12%
11–16	26.1%	1.09%
>16	57.3%	12.8%

CIN, Contrast-induced nephropathy; GFR, glomerular filtration rate. *Source:* From reference 37.

It has been known for many years that hydration is critical for prevention of contrast-induced nephropathy, and when furosemide-based intervention is compared with saline hydration, there is a negative effect of the furosemide-based intervention.[2,25]

Volume supplementation, therefore, is important and requires IV fluids for 12 hours pre-procedure and 12 hours post procedure.[35,44] Some protocols use 2 liters of normal saline within 12 hours before and after contrast media exposure. A protective effect of sodium bicarbonate has been demonstrated. A typical approach is to add 154 mEq/L of sodium bicarbonate in 5% dextrose in water and by adding 154 mL of 1,000 mEq/L sodium bicarbonate to 846 mL of 5% dextrose in water, diluting the dextrose concentration to 4.23%. In a randomized trial, only 1 of 60 patients treated with sodium bicarbonate developed contrast-induced nephropathy.[27] A recent systematic view showed benefit from *N*-acetylcysteine, theophylline, sodium bicarbonate and statins and, as mentioned above, increased possible harm risk with furosemide.[22]

Contrast osmolarity also may play a role, and the risk of developing acute renal failure is higher when patients receive an isoosmolar agent rather than a hypoosmolar agent.[24,31] In general, high osmolar contrast and ionic contrast increase the risk of contrast-induced nephropathy. There are many drugs and factors that can play an additional role, including metformin, anemia and blood loss, low hematocrit, the use of nonsteroidal anti-inflammatory drugs, intraarterial balloon pump hypotension, low serum albumin, hypercholesterolemia, and hypercalcemia.[37,38,43]

Gadolinium is a commonly used contrast medium to image the brain and its vessels, but it is excreted unchanged by the kidney. There are several hundred documented cases of nephrogenic systemic fibrosis, and many patients have died from this complication. The disorder appears as fibrotic nodules gradually spread over extremities and trunk; but fibrosis also involves lungs, myocardium, pleura, and pericardium.[10,14,34] A particular concern is with patients with prior renal failure (even low-grade kidney disease), which has resulted in an FDA blackbox warning (the actual risk may be 5% in dialysis patients). Radiologists do not administer gadolinium in patients with a GFR <30 mL/min per 1.73 m^2 or when they undergo dialysis.[34]

Nephrotoxicity can also be a result of drug use in acutely ill neurologic patients who have become critically ill.[9,33] Risk factors for nephrotoxicity include older age, diabetes mellitus, chronic kidney disease, malignancy, and acute factors such as sepsis, volume depletion, acute cardiac failure, hypotension, complex major surgery, trauma, and even mechanical ventilation.[33] Table 10.3 shows causes of drug-induced acute kidney injury in the intensive care unit.

The relationship between vancomycin and nephrotoxicity is well established and quite problematic due to the common use of vancomycin in hospitals. Vancomycin use has increased due to increase in methicillin-resistant *Staphylococcus aureus*, and over time there may have been a rise in average vancomycin minimum inhibitory concentration. In some instances, vancomycin is administered while, frankly, patients could be easily treated with methicillin.[40] Vancomycin trough concentrations of more than 50 mcg/mL is a risk factor for nephrotoxicity. When these concentrations are present, the risk is increased three-fold.[6]

If kidney failure occurs in any of these circumstances, patients become oliguric. A high dose of IV furosemide (15–20 mg/h) may be needed to obtain a negative fluid balance. In some patients, pulmonary edema occurs and then transient dialysis may be needed to remove excess fluids. Management is particularly difficult when a polyuric phase occurs, and creatinine may transiently increase with use of diuretics. Contrast nephropathy usually improves within days.

Equally important is dosing of antimicrobials in nephrotoxicity and some cause neurotoxicity (amphotericin B, metronidazole, penicillin derivatives). There has been renewed interest in toxicity due to cefepime. Cefepime may result in neurotoxicity even after a renal-adjusted dosing.[13] All β-lactam antibiotics can cause neurotoxicity. Cefepime is usually used in patients with febrile neutropenia and has very uncommon side effects, although neurotoxicity presenting

Table 10.3 **Drug-Induced Acute Kidney Injury in Critically Ill Patients**

Hemodynamic acute kidney injury
Nonsteroidal anti-inflammatory drugs (NSAIDs)
RAAS inhibitors
Calcineurin inhibitors (cyclosporine, tacrolimus)
Vasopressors
Acute tubular necrosis
Radiocontrast
Nephrotoxic antimicrobials
Osmotic nephropathy
Hydroxyethyl starch (HES)
Intravenous immunoglobulin (IVIG containing sucrose)
Crystal nephropathy
Highly active antiretroviral therapy (HAART)
Acyclovir
Ciprofloxacin
Sodium phosphate purgatives
Acute interstitial nephritis
Antibiotics (β-lactams, sulfa-based, quinolones)
Proton pump inhibitors, H_2 antagonists
Antiepileptic drugs

Abbreviations: H_2, histamine-2; NSAIDs, nonsteroidal anti-inflammatory drugs; RAAS, renin-angiotensin-aldosterone system. *Source:* From reference 33.

as nonconvulsive status epilepticus has been increasingly reported. The manifestations of cefepime neurotoxicity can be dramatic, with generalized myoclonus, sudden muteness, and stupor with an EEG correlate of epileptic discharges. Discontinuation of cefepime IV and loading with phenytoin is usually successful in management. In some patients—including in our experience—treatment with midazolam IV to control seizures may be needed before cefepime is excreted in patients with prior renal failure. Unfortunately, routine assays for serum cefepime concentrations are not available but cefepime levels can be considered increased in any patient who has a renal insufficiency.

DRUG-INDUCED ANGIOEDEMA

Orolingual angioedema is a rapid progressive complication that may need emergent airway management with intubation or even cricothyrotomy. The most common drugs that cause angioedema are tissue plasminogen activator (tPA) and angiotensin-converting-enzyme (ACE) inhibitors (even after years of use).[3,12] Angioedema is produced by increased plasma kinins. An increase in bradykinin has major properties and increases vascular permeability, resulting in swelling of lips and posterior of pharynx. When the edema involves only the interior tongue and lips, intubation is not necessary. However, patients with laryngeal or hypopharyngeal involvement or patients with involvement of the palate, floor of the mouth, or oropharynx this situation may progress very rapidly. Intubation at a later stage is very problematic. A skilled intubator is necessary for symptomatic patients when edema involves the posterior parts, and flexible fiber-optic airway inspection might be needed with nasotracheal intubation because supraglottic edema can obscure the glottic view. Treatment should always involve epinephrine (EpiPen auto-injector) in addition to antihistamines and corticosteroids. Patients are best treated with 0.3 mg intramuscular epinephrine, 10 mg IV dexamethasone, and 50 mg IV diphenhydramine. Two units of fresh frozen plasma (resulting in degrading of bradykinesis) can be a very successful additional treatment.[21] Swelling subsides over 72 hours but may take several more days.

DRUG-INDUCED HYPERPYREXIA SYNDROMES

Hyperpyrexia syndromes are very rare and despite high fever are easy to miss as such. The most common of these rare syndromes are reactions to anticholinergics, antidopaminergics, selective serotonin reuptake inhibitors, and tricyclic antidepressants.

Best known is neuroleptic malignant syndrome, but it occurs in less than 1% of patients taking neuroleptic drugs. The most commonly implicated neuroleptic drugs are haloperidol and fluphenazine, but all of the atypical antipsychotic drugs (clozapine, risperidone, and olanzapine) have been implicated. The least considered are metoclopramide and promethazine. High dose and a reaction to the first dose are common scenarios, as are recent dose escalations of the aforementioned drugs. Concomitant use of lithium may increase the risk.

Agitated delirium, mutism, and catatonia are prominent early signs, followed by muscular rigidity and high fever ("warm and stiff"). Patients are tachycardic and may be tachypneic with some degree of sweating. The clinical diagnosis is supported by marked increase in serum creatine kinase (CK) up to 10,000 IU/L and even much higher. Fever and dehydration will lead to other laboratory abnormalities including hypocalcemia, hypomagnesemia, and hypernatremia. Serum creatinine may rise quickly if rhabdomyolysis is not treated with high fluid intake.

Other related disorders are serotonin syndrome and the exceedingly rare syndrome malignant hyperthermia. Serotonin syndrome presents very similarly to malignant neuroleptic syndrome, but myoclonus (characteristically in the legs), is typical and almost even pathognomonic. On further examination the patient has prominent clonus in rigid extremities.

Treatment for each of these disorders is to stop the causative agent and to proceed with early rehydration, electrolyte replacement, treatment of cardiac arrhythmias in extreme manifestations, and treatment of hypertension, preferably with clonidine. Cooling with cooling pads is essential. Dantrolene (1 mg/kg IV followed by repeated doses up to 10 mg/kg IV) is rapidly effective but is associated with some rebound if not followed by a gradual taper in a week. Bromocriptine (2.5 mg orally every 6 hours) may be used next to dantrolene and also may need at least 7–10 days of treatment to avoid a relapse.[4,26, 42]

Drug Withdrawal Symptoms

Abrupt discontinuation of drugs in any patient may lead to a serious withdrawal syndrome. Many patients with an acute ischemic stroke are allowed a "permissive hypertension," but sudden withdrawal of antihypertensives may lead to overshoot of blood pressure. This applies to β-blockers and clonidine allowing suddenly increased sympathetic activity. New signs are a sudden tachycardia, new atrial fibrillation with rapid ventricular response, and new angina pectoris, and serum troponin as a result of demand ischemia may "bump" transiently.[18]

Sudden withdrawal of antiparkinson medication (L-dopa or dopamine agonist therapy) may cause a syndrome identical to neuroleptic malignant syndrome but it is called parkinsonism—hyperpyrexia syndrome. The disorder is also best treated with dantrolene among other measures used in treatment of neuroleptic malignant syndrome.[11,16,30]

The most serious and life-threatening syndrome is baclofen withdrawal. The major problems are not with oral medication but intrathecal pump dysfunction. Withdrawal of baclofen occurs 12–24 hours after medication is stopped or drastically reduced. Tachycardia, hypertension, tachypnea, rigidity are common. Progressive confusion precedes an agitated delirium. The treatment is difficult. Large oral doses (>120 mg daily in 6 divided doses) are needed, but oral baclofen may not be well absorbed. An intrathecal bolus through an intrathecally placed catheter may be the only solution, followed by pump replacement. Propofol (5–15 mg/h) is an effective treatment, as is IV benzodiazepine in high doses. Dantrolene or cyproheptadine—a central acting muscle relaxants are commonly used. Tizanidine (8–12 mg/day total in divided doses) has also been proven effective.[1,28,36]

DRUG INTERACTIONS

Drug interactions are expected and are a result of commonly used polypharmacy. Drug interactions can lead to medical complications; best known are hypokalemia, hypotension, hypertension, and cardiac arrhythmias. With current computer databases and warning programs, hospital pharmacists often identify these drug interactions early and they can explain the changed pharmacokinetics.

Some drugs inhibit the metabolism of benzodiazepines, increasing their effect and causing more-than-expected drowsiness. Calcium channel blockers (cytochrome P450 inhibitor, erythromycin, fluconazole) all prolong sedation.

The class of drugs about which there is the greatest unfamiliarity among physicians is antiepileptic drugs.[5,17,19] Common interactions are shown in Table 10.4. There are some simple rules to remember. Most antiepileptic drugs decrease international normalized ratio (INR), and valproate increases INR in patients receiving warfarin. Many antiepileptic drugs decrease the effect of commonly used drugs such as corticosteroids and tricyclic antidepressants. Sudden discontinuation of most antiepileptic drugs can result in marked increase in INR and lead to bleeding complications.

ADVERSE EFFECTS OF OTHER THERAPEUTIC INTERVENTIONS

Several other nonpharmaceutical therapeutic interventions in acute neurologic patients should be addressed. Plasma exchange is commonly used in Guillain-Barré syndrome, myasthenia gravis, fulminant forms of multiple sclerosis, acute disseminated encephalomyelitis, autoimmune encephalitis, and paraneoplastic manifestations.[8] Plasma exchange requires a high-flow catheter to exchange approximately 2.5–3 liters of plasma replaced with small amount of plasma, large amounts of 5% albumin, and some heparin in approximately one hour. Red blood cell loss must not be more than 25 mL after one series of five

Table 10.4 **Antiepileptic Drug Interactions in Acutely Ill Neurologic Patients**

Valproic Acid and Warfarin
Mode of action: especially with loading dose. Drug displacement in protein-binding site, with a high loading dose reaching in higher serum level may likely displace warfarin from total plasma-binding site.
Phenytoin and Fluconazole
Mode of action: Fluconazole inhibits phenytoin metabolism and may increase phenytoin level up to four times. Serum concentration monitoring with a reduction in phenytoin dosage is warranted.
Valproic Acid and Carbapenems
Mode of action: The exact mechanism is unknown. Carbapenems, especially meropenem, may inhibit valproic acid absorption. Meropenem may accelerate the renal excretion and may result in low valproic acid serum level and increase risk of seizures. Additionally, carbapenems lower seizure threshold.

Source: From Wijdicks and Rabinstein. *Neurocritical Care.* New York, Oxford University Press, 2012.

total plasma exchanges. Complications are substantially more common with fresh frozen plasma exchanges than with albumin. A serious anaphylaxis is very uncommon, however more common (as mentioned earlier) in patients on ACE inhibitors. Hypotension is uncommon and seen only in patients who may have more than 200 mL negative balance after full exchange. Fluid bolus with normal saline is usually very effective, but persistent hypotension may have to be treated by placement in Trendelenburg's position and administration of a bolus of albumin. A transfusion-related acute lung injury (Chapter 8) is very uncommon, but mortality may reach 10%.

A more common side effect of plasma exchange is a reduction of serum potassium; this may be substantial and more than 25 % from baseline value. A mild metabolic acidosis is also a known side effect of plasma exchange and is citrate related. Other commonly reported side effects are vasovagal reactions, hypovolemia, allergic reactions, hemolysis from kinking in the tubing; and almost never, air embolization.

IVIG is used in Guillain-Barré syndrome, myasthenia gravis, inflammatory myopathies, and autoimmune encephalitis. The side effects are quite minor but may involve acute renal failure in formulas with high sucrose content. Aseptic meningitis is very uncommon (only a few well-documented case reports), but headache may occur in one of five patients treated.[32] Other incidental side effects are transient fever, chills, urticaria, arthralgia, and hyperglycemia.[32] Pseudohyponatremia can be due to a laboratory artifact when an automated laboratory method does not correct for increased protein concentrations.

Putting It All Together

- Many noncardiac drugs may cause EKG changes with potential for life-threatening arrhythmias
- Protecting the kidney is important when considering computed tomography with iodinated contrast or magnetic resonance angiogram with gadolinium
- Drug interactions are many; only a few are consequential and usually occur with antiepileptic drugs.
- Drugs can cause angioedema, resulting in rapid loss of airway patency
- Drugs can cause serious hyperpyrexia syndromes but also withdrawal of parkinsonian drugs

References

1. Ackland GL, Fox R. Low-dose propofol infusion for controlling acute hyperspasticity after withdrawal of intrathecal baclofen therapy. *Anesthesiology* 2005;103:663–665.

2. Bader BD, Berger ED, Heede MB, et al. What is the best hydration regimen to prevent contrast media-induced nephrotoxicity? *Clin Nephrol* 2004;62:1–7.

3. Banerji A, Clark S, Blanda M, et al. Multicenter study of patients with angiotensin-converting enzyme inhibitor-induced angioedema who present to the emergency department. *Ann Allergy Asthma Immunol* 2008;100:327–332.

4. Berman BD. Neuroleptic malignant syndrome. *Neurohospitalist* 2011;1:41–47.

5. Bertsche T, Pfaff J, Schiller P, et al. Prevention of adverse drug reactions in intensive care patients by personal intervention based on an electronic clinical decision support system. *Intensive Care Med* 2010;36:665–672.

6. Bosso JA, Nappi J, Rudisill C, et al. Relationship between vancomycin trough concentrations and nephrotoxicity: a prospective multicenter trial. *Antimicrob Agents Chemother* 2011;55:5475–5479.

7. Buckley MS, Leblanc JM, Cawley MJ. Electrolyte disturbances associated with commonly prescribed medications in the intensive care unit. *Crit Care Med* 2010;38:S253–S264.

8. Chhibber V, Weinstein R. Evidence-based review of therapeutic plasma exchange in neurologic disorders. *Seminars Dialysis* 2012;25:132–139.

9. Dennen P, Douglas IS, Anderson R. Acute kidney injury in the intensive care unit: an update and primer for the intensivist. *Crit Care Med* 2010;38:261–275.

10. Evenepoel P, Zeegers M, Segaert S, et al. Nephrogenic fibrosing dermopathy: a novel, disabling disorder in patients with renal failure. *Nephrol Dial Transplant* 2004;19:469–473.

11. Fricchione G, Mann SC, Caroff SN. Catatonia, lethal catatonia, and neuroleptic malignant syndrome. *Psychiatr Ann* 2000;30:347–355.

12. Fugate JE, Kalimullah EA, Wijdicks EF. Angioedema after tPA: what neurointensivists should know. *Neurocrit Care* 2012;16:440–443.

13. Gangireddy VG, Mitchell LC, Coleman T. Cefepime neurotoxicity despite renal adjusted dosing. *Scand J Infect Dis* 2011;43:827–829.

14. Gibson SE, Farver CF, Prayson RA. Multiorgan involvement in nephrogenic fibrosing dermopathy: an autopsy case and review of the literature. *Arch Pathol Lab Med* 2006;130:209–212.

15. Gitler B, Berger LS, Buffa SD. Torsades de pointes induced by erythromycin. *Chest* 1994;105:368–372.

16. Granner MA, Wooten GF. Neuroleptic malignant syndrome or Parkinsonism hyperpyrexia syndrome. *Semin Neurol* 1991;11:228–235.

17. Guthrie SK, Stoysich AM, Bader G, Hilleman DE. Hypothesized interaction between valproic acid and warfarin. *J Clin Psychopharmacol* 1995;15:138–139.

18. Houston MC. Abrupt cessation of treatment in hypertension: consideration of clinical features, mechanisms, prevention and management of the discontinuation syndrome. *Am Heart J* 1981;102:415–430.

19. Juurlink DN, Mamdani M, Kopp A, Laupacis A, Redelmeier DA. Drug-drug interactions among elderly patients hospitalized for drug toxicity. *JAMA* 2003;289:1652–1658.

20. Kane-Gill SL, Jacobi J, Rothschild JM. Adverse drug events in intensive care units: risk factors, impact, and the role of team care. *Crit Care Med* 2010;38:S83–S89.

21. Karim MY, Masood A. Fresh-frozen plasma as a treatment for life-threatening ACE-inhibitor angioedema. *J Allergy Clin Immunol* 2002;109:370–371.

22. Kwok CS, Pang CL, Yeong JK, Loke YK. Measures used to treat contrast-induced nephropathy: overview of reviews. *Br J Radiol* 2013;86:20120272.

23. Li EC, Esterly JS, Pohl S, Scott SD, McBride BF. Drug-induced QT-interval prolongation: considerations for clinicians. *Pharmacotherapy* 2010;30:684–701.

24. Liss P, Persson PB, Hansell P, Lagerqvist B. Renal failure in 57 925 patients undergoing coronary procedures using iso-osmolar or low-osmolar contrast media. *Kidney Int* 2006;70:1811–1817.

25. Marenzi G, Ferrari C, Marana I, et al. Prevention of contrast nephropathy by furosemide with matched hydration: the MYTHOS (Induced Diuresis With Matched Hydration Compared to Standard Hydration for Contrast Induced Nephropathy Prevention) trial. *JACC Cardiovasc Interv* 2012;5:90–97.

26. McAllen KJ, Schwartz DR. Adverse drug reactions resulting in hyperthermia in the intensive care unit. *Crit Care Med* 2010;38:S244–S252.

27. Merten GJ, Burgess WP, Gray LV, et al. Prevention of contrast-induced nephropathy with sodium bicarbonate: a randomized controlled trial. *JAMA* 2004;291:2328–2334.

28. Meythaler JM, Roper JF, Brunner RC. Cyproheptadine for intrathecal baclofen withdrawal. *Arch Phys Med Rehabil* 2003;84:638–642.

29. Mitcheson JS, Chen J, Lin M, Culberson C, Sanguinetti MC. A structural basis for drug-induced long QT syndrome. *Proc Natl Acad Sci USA* 2000;97:12329–12333.

30. Newman EJ, Grosset DG, Kennedy PG. The parkinsonism-hyperpyrexia syndrome. *Neurocrit Care* 2009;10:136–140.

31. Panwar B, Johnson VA, Patel M, Balkovetz DF. Risk of vancomycin-induced nephrotoxicity in the population with chronic kidney disease. *Am J Med Sci* 2013;345:396–369.

32. Patwa HS, Chaudhry V, Katzberg H, Rae-Grant AD, So YT. Evidence-based guideline: intravenous immunoglobulin in the treatment of neuromuscular disorders: report of the Therapeutics and Technology Assessment Subcommittee of the American Academy of Neurology. *Neurology* 2012;78:1009–1015.

33. Perazella MA. Drug use and nephrotoxicity in the intensive care unit. *Kidney Int* 2012;81:1172–1178.

34. Perez-Rodriguez J, Lai S, Ehst BD, Fine DM, Bluemke DA. Nephrogenic systemic fibrosis: incidence, associations, and effect of risk factor assessment—report of 33 cases. *Radiology* 2009;250:371–377.

35. Richenberg J. How to reduce nephropathy following contrast-enhanced CT: A lesson in policy implementation. *Clin Radiol* 2012;67:1136–1145.

36. Ross JC, Cook AM, Stewart GL, Fahy BG. Acute intrathecal baclofen withdrawal: a brief review of treatment options. *Neurocrit Care* 2011;14:103–108.

37. Rundback JH, Nahl D, Yoo V. Contrast-induced nephropathy. *J Vasc Surg* 2011;54:575–579.

38. Schetz M, Dasta J, Goldstein S, Golper T. Drug-induced acute kidney injury. *Curr Opin Crit Care* 2005;11:555–565.

39. Smithburger PL, Seybert AL, Armahizer MJ, Kane-Gill SL. QT prolongation in the intensive care unit: commonly used medications and the impact of drug-drug interactions. *Expert Opin Drug Saf* 2010;9:699–712.

40. Steinkraus G, White R, Friedrich L. Vancomycin MIC creep in non-vancomycin-intermediate *Staphylococcus aureus* (VISA), vancomycin-susceptible clinical methicillin-resistant *S. aureus* (MRSA) blood isolates from 2001-05. *J Antimicrob Chemother* 2007;60:788–794.

41. Straus SM, Kors JA, De Bruin ML, et al. Prolonged QTc interval and risk of sudden cardiac death in a population of older adults. *J Am Coll Cardiol* 2006;47:362–367.

42. Strawn JR, Keck PE Jr, Caroff SN. Neuroleptic malignant syndrome. *Am J Psychiatry* 2007;164:870–876.

43. Taber SS, Mueller BA. Drug-associated renal dysfunction. *Crit Care Clin* 2006;22:357–374.

44. Trivedi HS, Moore H, Nasr S, et al. A randomized prospective trial to assess the role of saline hydration on the development of contrast nephrotoxicity. *Nephron Clin Pract* 2003;93:C29–34.

45. Yap YG, Camm AJ. Drug induced QT prolongation and torsades de pointes. *Heart* 2003;89:1363–1372.

Index

Page numbers followed by 'f' refer to figures.